5:2

diet

igloobooks

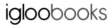

Published in 2015
by Igloo Books Ltd
Cottage Farm
Sywell
NN6 0BJ
www.igloobooks.com

Cover image featured on this book is courtesy of Getty Images © Getty Images
Food photography and recipe development: Photocuisine UK
Additional images supplied courtesy of Thinkstock, Getty Images

Written by Alison Marlow

FIR003 0215
2 4 6 8 10 9 7 5 3 1
ISBN 978-1-78440-149-8

Printed and manufactured in China

The information and advice contained in this book
are intended as a general guide. Neither the author
nor the publishers can be held responsible for claims
arising from the inappropriate use of any remedy or
exercise regime. The author and publisher advise the
reader to check with a doctor before changing diet
and undertaking any course of treatment or exercise.

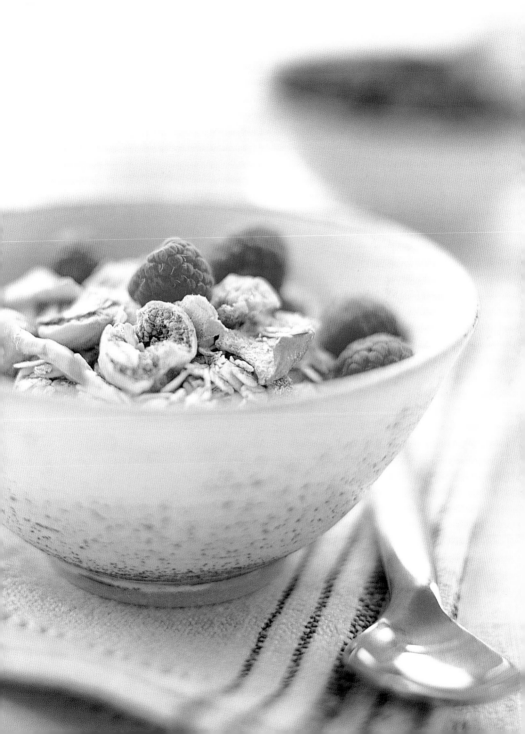

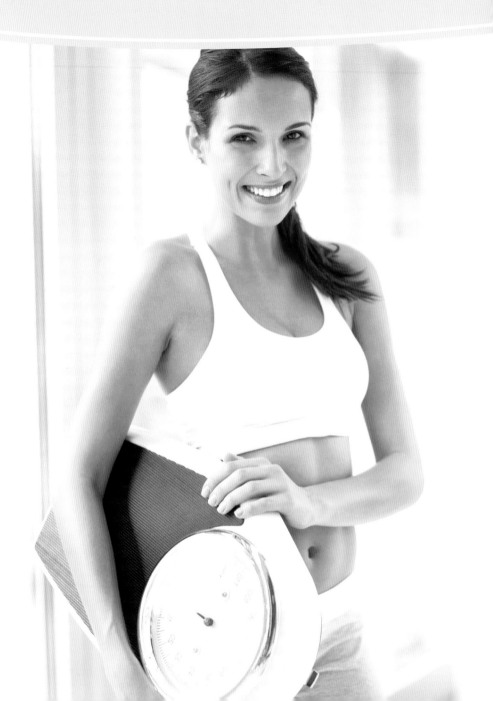

Contents

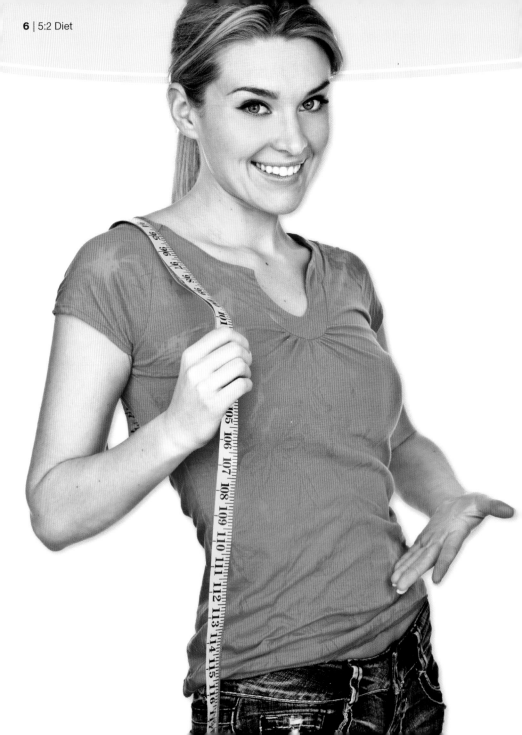

Introduction

When you want to lose a few pounds you want to do it as effortlessly as possible, right? You don't want to have to buy special foods or branded goods that involve counting units or restrict you from eating the things that you love every single day of the week.

And most of all, you don't want it to take up all of your time. We've all met diet bores – the people who talk about their weight loss plan all the time. You know the sort. They reel off every morsel that's passed their lips today – and then tell you exactly what they're going to eat later, down to the exact number of peas. And the next day, they admit that they didn't quite manage it and start all over again.

This plan is different. It is also incredibly simple. For five days of the week, you can eat whatever you like within the recommended guidelines of up to 2000 calories a day for women, or 2500 for men. On two other days, you restrict yourself to 500 calories (600 for men). That's it. This 5:2 combination of five days off, two days on gives you a gradual weight loss that is easy to manage for as long as you want to lose weight.

Intermittent fasting has been around for centuries – now is the time to make it work for you!

The Science Of Fasting

The idea of using fasting days to lose weight first reached the general public via a BBC Horizon documentary called Eat, Fast and Live Longer, shown on television in August 2012.

It is based on the principle called Intermittent Fasting (IF) where you eat normally on certain days and fast on others. It has its roots in the days of early man, when hunter-gatherers would go for lengthy fast periods while searching for food.

The theory is that being hungry made man's brain sharper – and therefore he was better able to hunt the food needed to stave off hunger pangs. Back in the days of cave-dwellers, it would have been quite normal for people to go hungry for several hours on the trot, before feasting on whatever they managed to catch. Early man would have naturally practised intermittent fasting but would probably never have gone more than a day before refuelling.

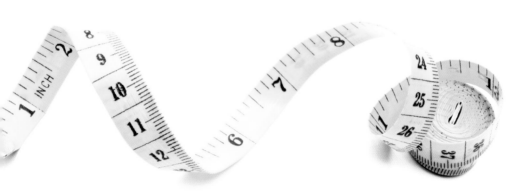

Fans of this way of eating claim that as well as helping people lose weight, the 5:2 diet can offer other health benefits including increased life-span, protection from certain diseases and improved cognitive function. Currently, there is a limited body of evidence about intermittent fasting, but as this way of eating becomes more popular there is likely to be more scientific research into the area.

There have been some studies into the effectiveness of the 5:2 diet. In one study* in 2010 researchers did discover that women on a 5:2 diet achieved similar levels of weight loss as those achieved by women on a calorie-controlled diet.

They also found reductions in some biological indicators or biomarkers that suggest a reduction in the risk of developing chronic conditions such as type 2 diabetes.

Another study** in 2012 suggested that the 5:2 diet model may help reduce the risk of some obesity-related cancers, such as breast cancer.

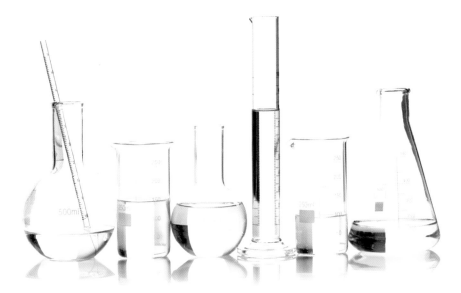

*Harvie, M. *et al*. (2010) 'The effects of intermittent or continuous energy restriction on weight loss and metabolic disease risk markers: A randomised trial in young overweight women', *International Journal of Obesity*.
**Harvie, M. and Howell, A. (2012) 'Energy restriction and the prevention of breast cancer', Cambridge University Press.

The Ancient Art Of Fasting

Fasting is not a modern invention

For thousands of years, fasting – or abstaining from food, or certain types of food – has been used as a way to cleanse the body, open the mind and give the faster an increased sense of wellbeing. It has been observed on all continents and in many religions and cultures.

Even before that, early man would have fasted as part of every day life. Like animals, he would have had fasting enforced on him at some point – during times of stress, or illness or food shortage. We all know people who go off their food at the smallest sign of uneasiness. That tendency to stop eating for a while is the body's way of seeking to rest, balance and conserve energy till it's needed most.

Fasting has its formal origins in serving the metaphysical needs of people. In its earliest usage it was thought to be good for purifying the soul for penance, mental clarity and redemption. This was when it was used for religious or cultural reasons rather than as a weight loss programme.

The roots – religious

Fasting has long been used in many religions, from Hinduism, Islam and Buddhism to Christianity, Mormonism and Judaism.

It is seen as an important part of religious practice, with many fasting days and periods throughout the calendar. Depending on the religion followed, certain foods, drinks and other substances are limited or avoided.

In Islam, Muslims fast for one month each year during Ramadan. This action serves as a reminder of the time when the Qur'an was revealed to Muhammad after he fasted. The aim is to prove devotion to Allah as well as discipline and conscientiousness of faith. In Islam, fasting is one of the so-called five pillars of Islam.

Fasting also has its place in both Jewish and Christian religions. Moses fasted for 40 days on Mount Sinai. Jesus fasted and prayed for 40 days in the wilderness. Today, Christians mark the Passion of Christ with Lent, a 40-day period before Easter when parishioners are encouraged to give something up for Lent and donate whatever money they save to charity.

The Jewish calendar has six days of fasting. The most well-known and most important is Yom Kippur, the day of reconciliation.

In ancient Greece, there was ritual fasting. This took place during the Eleusinian Mysteries to honour Demeter, the goddess of fertility. And other notable names, including Cicero, were known to have fasted in a bid to increase their mental performance.

And as recently as the 20th century, Mahatma Gandhi, the father of the Indian independence movement, popularised fasting across India and around the world as a means of promoting passive resistance.

He went on a fast on behalf of the 'untouchables' in India. And he also publicly fasted for Hindus and Muslims to work peacefully side by side.
This very peaceful form of protest has been used by many people across the globe to make their point to the powers that be.

The roots – medical

Although fasting began for religious and cultural reasons, people rapidly recognised that it had some medical benefits.

Hippocrates believed that fasting had 'miraculous' healing powers. He used certain foods to treat specific ailments. Greek philosopher Plato was known to have fasted for mental and physical efficiency. They believed that fasting could heal the body and spirit.

Mathematician and philosopher Pythagoras asked his followers to stick to a strict 40-day fast as he felt it improved mental perception and creativity. Six hundred years later, Roman doctor Galen believed that fasting was an effective therapy for ensuring that bodily fluids were kept in equilibrium.

In the 11th century, Hildegard von Bingen recommended fasting as a remedy to treat various illnesses. And later on, during the 16th century, Paracelsus believed the body's functions could be correctly regulated by the use of fasting.

The roots – cultural

Many cultures have historically incorporated fasting into their way of life. Native American Indians would often fast prior to their sacred ceremonies. Fasting was often used as an offering to the Great Spirit.

Fasting would be used at different times throughout the year and also at important moments – such as the onset of puberty or prior to marriage. Native Americans believed that a fast cleansed both the mind and body, freeing them to understand omens or messages of good fortune from the Great Spirit.

Devotees of yoga also use fasting methods that date back thousands of years. Yogi Paramahansa Yogananda believed that fasting was a natural method of healing and even today the practice of Ayurveda includes fasting as a form of therapy.

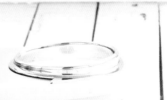

Why Fasting Works

Eating the 5:2 way can work for weight loss on many levels. If you go on a 'standard' weight loss diet, you need to cut down approximately 3,500 calories in order to lose a pound in weight. Reducing your daily calorie intake by 500 calories could mean that you would therefore lose one pound a week.

Eating plans like this where you are dieting all the time, can lead to feelings of deprivation and a tendency to slip. Anyone who has tried to diet 24/7 knows that it can be a long slog, especially with our hectic lifestyles where food seems to tempt us every step of the way.

With the 5:2 approach, you just need to get yourself into the mindset that you only have to cut right down for two days out of every seven. In reality, it's just one day of restricted eating before you can eat normally again. Many people find it comparatively easy to get through the fast days – they even find that they have no desire to splurge and scoff themselves on the other five days of the week.

And only 'being good' for two days out of a week is a much more manageable concept than feeling you have to watch what you're eating every single day in order to lose weight.

It can take you a few weeks to get into the 5:2 groove, but lots of people find that it works well for them.

It's easy to plan around your lifestyle too. Whereas 'full-time' dieting requires times when you are compromised by the food situations around you – birthday buffets, girls' nights out, festive parties – the 5:2 approach means you can pick your fast days around your schedule.

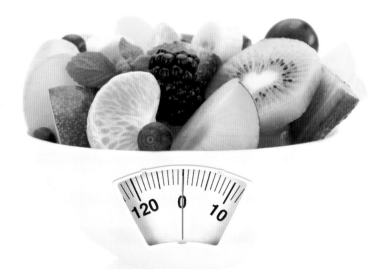

Easy to plan

You can choose your fast days to fit round you. That's the wonderful thing about the 5:2 diet – you tailor-make it to your way of life, your work and home commitments. It's just about the most personalised diet there can be. As you'll see from the meal ideas for fast days, there is so much flexibility to what you choose to eat and when you choose to eat it.

The only real rules are that you restrict yourself to 500 calories (600 for men) over two non-consecutive days of the week. The rest is up to you.

If you're worried that you'll be fine all day long and then get the bedtime munchies, restrict your food during the day and eat something later so that you don't go to bed feeling deprived.

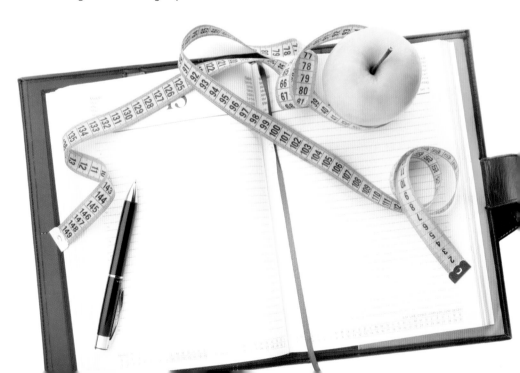

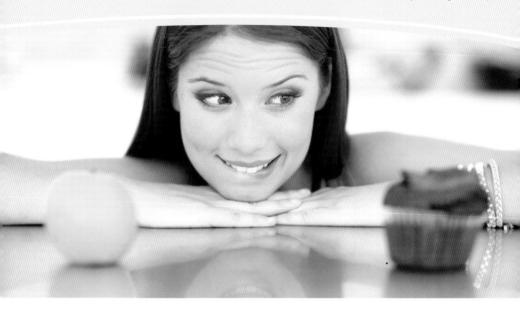

The 5:2 diet is good too, because, unless you want to shout it from the rooftops, people don't need to know that you're on a diet at all. And that can be good for many reasons. You don't have to listen to the diet saboteurs who tell you it'll never work, or that you don't need to lose weight anyway. You don't have to have the office diet bore try and talk you into trying another method instead. You can choose your fast days to be times when you'd have time to yourself anyway, and you can ensure that they don't clash with a day where you need to do lots of communal eating, such as a party or family get together.

The 5:2 diet even allows for things not going quite to plan. If for some reason, you get stuck in a situation where you simply can't avoid eating normal size portions – say, your boss insists on taking the team out for a pizza – then you can admit defeat and put off one of your two fasting days to later in the week.

And that's what makes the 5:2 diet so popular right now: it puts you in control. And as you're the one steering your own progress, you are much, much more likely to keep to it and lose those pounds you're longing to wave goodbye to!

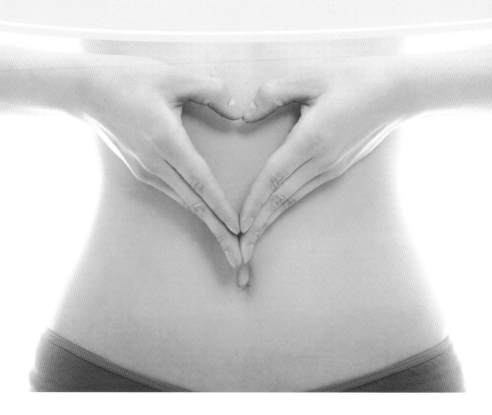

Health Benefits

You only have to lose a few pounds to recognise that shifting that excess fat can work wonders for your physical and mental health. Your clothes feel looser, your skin looks brighter and somehow you feel you can cope so much better with whatever life has to throw at you.

Getting to within your normal weight range offers many more benefits than just being able to fit into your old jeans.

There are also many general benefits associated with losing excess weight. If you're overweight or obese, you have a higher risk of such health conditions as:

- High blood pressure
- Heart disease
- Stroke
- Type 2 diabetes
- Some types of cancer
- Infertility
- Osteoarthritis
- Back pain
- Depression

Getting your weight back down to an acceptable level can help reduce the risks of developing many of the above conditions.

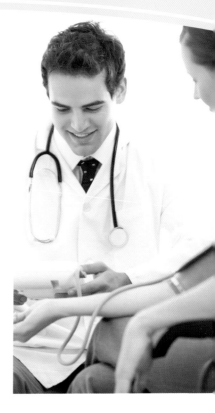

What is my ideal weight?

You can get five people of the same height together and they will all look different. There will be people with broad shoulders and others with tiny frames. That's why standard height/weight charts allow a fair few pounds of leeway. What's an ideal weight for one person might be way too low (or too high) for another.

GPs often use BMI as an indicator as to whether your weight falls into an acceptable category. BMI stands for Body Mass Index and is a simple mathematical calculation that can quickly establish if you are an appropriate weight.

It works as an excellent guide for most people. Others who have a very high proportion of lean muscle, such as rugby players and serious athletes, may find that their BMI makes them appear fatter as more of their body weight is muscle and not fat.

For your average office worker or parent though, BMI is a good way of finding out if your weight is within a healthy range. Broadly speaking, if your BMI comes out at 25 or over, then you're overweight. If it's over 30, you're classified as obese.

Grab a calculator to work out where you stand. First weigh yourself in kilogrammes (kg). Then divide your weight by your height in metres (m). Divide the answer by your height again to get your correct BMI. E.g: if you are 1.65 metres tall and weigh 75kg, the sum would be as follows:

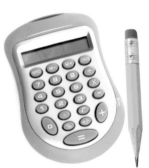

- 75 divided by 1.65 = 45.45

- Now divide by your height again
  45.45 divided by 1.65 = 27.54

- 27.54 is your BMI which would put you into the overweight category.

Using fasting as a weight loss regime in the 21st century is recognised to have a range of benefits including:

- Loss of excess weight
- Flushing toxins out of the body
- Cleansing the digestive system
- Clearing the mind
- Gaining energy
- Allowing the body time to rest and recover

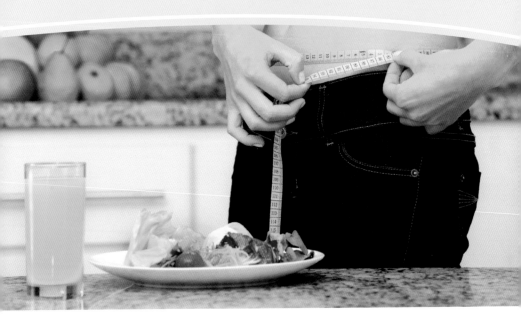

Many people who have tried the 5:2 diet sing its praises for the fact that severely restricting calories two days a week is actually quite manageable. And that is quite simply because your brain fully understands that it's for a very short space of time before 'normal' eating is resumed. It's a bit like waiting for a big birthday bash or counting the days down to Christmas. You know the end is in sight so that in itself makes whatever you're doing much more workable. And like dieting, if you can keep to the regime, you're bound to get results.

Another benefit is that you're less likely to crash and burn due to weeks and weeks of what you perceive to be daily deprivation. Because only two days are restricted, and the other five days of the week are not, it puts you in a psychologically stronger place to keep going.

And when you've reached your desired weight, using the 5:2 theory means that it's easy to go back on the diet if you slip up and gain a few pounds. You'll have already programmed your brain to accept this way of eating, so it can become a lifestyle choice, if that's what you want.

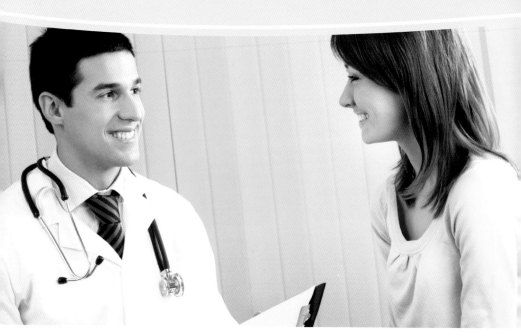

Is It Safe?

Even if you are in good general health and think you'll be fine to do the 5:2 diet, it's always a good idea to check with your GP first.

You shouldn't embark on this plan if:

• You are a child or teenager

• You are pregnant

• You are breast-feeding

• You have a history of eating disorders.

If you have type-2 diabetes or a lowered immune system, this diet might be right for you but you MUST check first with your doctor.

Before you start, stick a picture of yourself as you are now in this space – then in a few weeks' time you'll notice the difference!

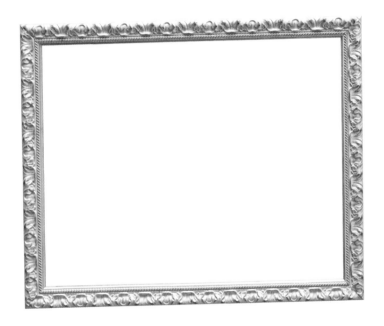

It's also a good idea to take your measurements. Sometimes, even if the weight loss appears to be slow, you'll nevertheless be losing those vital inches or centimetres.

Measurements now:

Bust/Chest

Waist

Hips

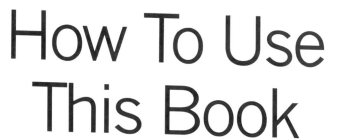

How To Use This Book

This book has been devised to help you stick to the 5:2 diet by offering lots of practical advice, recipe suggestions and handy hints.

Exactly how you choose to use your 500 calories a day on fast days (600 for men) is entirely up to you. We recognise that the more you can personalise your day's eating, the better your chance of success.

That's why we've come up with a selection of recipes for breakfast, brunch, lunch and dinner. We've also included a choice of snacks you might want to use and much more.

The best laid plans

Everyone knows that no two days are ever quite the same. And no matter how you might plan, things might not go exactly the way you expected them to. That's one of the advantages of the 5:2 diet – if, for some reason it becomes clear that your fasting day isn't working, then don't worry. Go back to your normal eating plan and pick another day to fast.

Which days do I choose?

That's entirely up to you, but you need to leave at least a day between your two fasting days. If you try and fast two days on the trot, this way of eating can start to feel like deprivation. And feelings of deprivation can lead you to throwing in the towel and heading for the pizza menu.

Your own weekly schedule is the best guide. Many people like to choose Monday as a fasting day (after a bit of weekend indulgence) and then Thursday, but whatever's right for you is the answer. You won't necessarily choose the same two fasting days each week either. For example, if you know you have a birthday celebration to attend, or a particularly stressful meeting on the cards, then don't fast on those days.

How will I feel?

Five hundred calories is obviously quite a severe restriction on what you'd normally eat, but most people say they find it relatively easy to manage. When you first start the 5:2 diet, you will probably get a few hunger pangs as your body adjusts. Occasionally, people might get a mild headache or the occasional bout of feeling dizzy. If this happens to you, take things steadily and don't over-exert yourself. Ensure you drink plenty of liquids so that you don't get dehydrated.

What To Eat And When

The 5:2 diet is just about the most tailor-made diet there is. You choose what you eat and when you eat it. On those two fasting days, the only real rules you follow are your own.

Fast days

On each fast day, you are allowed 500 calories (600 for men). You want those calories to offer you a good range of nutrients and be filling enough to get you through to the next day.

It can be tempting to go out and buy a 500-calorie bar of chocolate and be done with it. But there's no need to do that – that's the advantage of 5:2. There's no need to feel deprived when you know you can eat normally again tomorrow.

On the 5:2 diet you need to look quite carefully at the foods you choose to eat on the fasting days. Picking sensibly can reduce feelings of hunger and ensure that you get to the end of the day without cracking and diving for the biscuit tin.

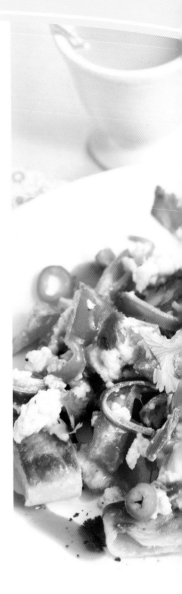

Some people choose to have their entire calorie allowance in one meal. While that is possible it does also require a good dollop of willpower. You could have a hearty breakfast of 500 calories that keeps you going all day, but then what do you do when you hit a hard hunger attack 10 hours later and have no calories left?

One of the best options it to split your calorie allowance, starting with a small breakfast, brunch or lunch, and then having the rest of your calories in the evening. Eating late afternoon or evening can give you a feeling of satisfaction and prevent the chance of you waking up with hunger pangs during the night.

Non-fast days

Treat these as ordinary eating days and aim to eat no more than the recommended daily allowance of 2000 calories for women (2500 for men). You may think you're going to want to eat lots after a fast day, but you'll probably find that you're actually more thoughtful and considered about what you eat. Choose plenty of wholegrain cereals, fresh fruit and vegetables, lean meat and calcium rich products such as low-fat cheese and semi-skimmed milk.

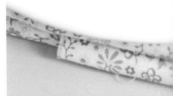

How To Fast

Which days do I fast?

That's entirely up to you. Just make sure that you don't fast two days on the trot. Many people like to choose Monday and then pick another day that suits them. Try to choose days when there aren't too many demands placed on you. For example, don't fast on a day when you have a 200-mile drive ahead, or if you have a job interview. Ideally fast days should be days where there is nothing unusual planned, just a simple, calm, straightforward day.

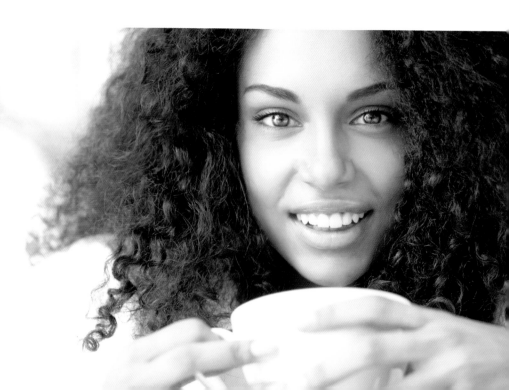

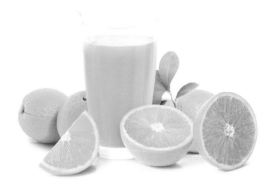

When do I eat on my fast days?

Really it's entirely up to you! Maybe you're one of those people who don't care to eat much in the evening – then choose to eat most of your calories at lunch? Perhaps you can't get out of bed without breakfast to tempt you – then have something light to have you throwing off the covers!

Over the next few pages, we've included plenty of ideas for meals to tempt your taste buds on your fast days. You might find it best to try some of these as you get used to your new way of eating, but there are bound to be recipes of your own you're going to want to include in your fast day plans.

Some people choose to eat a small breakfast and then stick to plenty of low-calorie drinks, such as water, tea and coffee throughout the day, saving up most of their calories for an evening meal.

Others find that they can happily manage without breakfast – relying on low-calorie drinks – until much later on in the morning. Then they might have a light snack followed by something a little more filling later on.

Our recipe ideas will give you plenty of inspiration about what to eat and when. Remember, it may take a few fast days for you to work out what's right for you.

Splitting the days

Make sure your two fast days are spread over the week and not back-to-back. The aim of the 5:2 diet is that your two fast days are intermingled between standard eating days – not squashed together. You don't have to stick to the same two days each week. Just pick the days that are best for you – that might mean a Wednesday and Saturday one week, and a Monday and Friday the following one.

Keep a record

When taking part in a weight loss regime, it's always a good idea to keep a record of what you've eaten and when. Even better, keep a note of your mood at the time as this can often pin-point times when you want to eat simply because you're bored or fed up. The diary pages in this book will help you keep track.

Stay busy

There are going to be times on fast days when you will feel peckish and have already used up your daily calorie allowance. One of the best things to do when hunger strikes is to do something to take your mind off it.

- Take a warm, bubble bath.

- Start a new project – treat yourself to some wool and get knitting. Anything that keeps your fingers busy is great news.

- Try painting watercolours.

- Have a clear out of your bedroom cupboards. De-cluttering is great for the mood and makes the time fly.

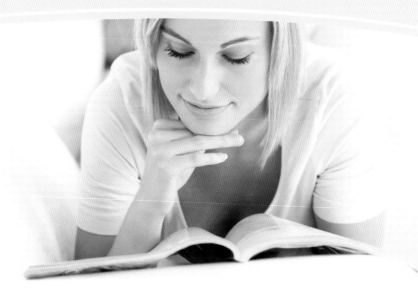

- Treat yourself to a magazine – not one that's crammed with pictures of cake though.

- Go for a long stroll with or without the dog.

- Have a long girlie catch-up with a mate you've not seen for ages.

- Go to bed a bit earlier. Take a good book with you and lose yourself in a great romance or thriller.

Early days

As with anything new, the early days of a new diet regime can be the toughest. This is the time when you have to get used to a new way of eating, and there will be times when you feel uncertain or unsure about whether you're eating the right thing at the right time.

You'll also probably be feeling pretty happy right now – at your decision to lose weight, about the fact that there are plenty of lovely dishes to enjoy on fast days. And even better, the fact that you know that if you stick to your 500 calories on two days, you can relax on the other five!

How To Eat

No point beating about the bush – on fast days you're not going to eat much at all. That's why it's really important to eat what you like. Don't pick meals containing ingredients you hate – for example, if you've always loathed cottage cheese, there's no point in adding it to your fast day. Eating stuff you dislike is only going to make you want to throw in the towel!

Make your meals as interesting as possible. Follow these tips for maximum success:

• On fast days, ensure your meals include some protein as protein rich foods can help keep you feeling satisfied for longer. Protein foods include fish, lean meats and poultry, eggs, low fat milk and cheese.

• Weigh and measure everything.

• Take a good multi-vitamin supplement to make sure you're not missing out on essential vitamins.

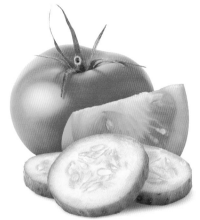

• Add lots of leafy vegetables to your fast days - try cabbage, kale and spring greens or go for salad veggies like rocket, fresh spinach and lamb's lettuce. Adding extra low-calorie vegetables like these can help keep you full and add vital fibre to your day.

- Make salad foods your friend. Not only does salad add lots of fibre it also makes small meals look bigger and more vibrant. Try grating carrot and mixing with rocket and red pepper for a real traffic light of a side dish!

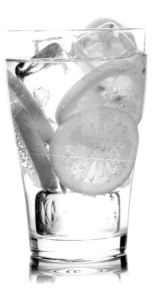

- Drink plenty. Fresh water is best. Add a squeeze of fresh lemon for extra zing. Other low-calorie drinks include tea, coffee, herbal teas, and low-calorie fruit squashes and diet drinks.

- Cook in a non-stick pan to avoid having to use fat. Add a little water if need be.

- Use skimmed milk and very low-fat yoghurt options.

- Avoid alcohol on fast days. Alcohol supplies empty calories and when you're only having 500 you want to use them all for food.

- Add spices to your food – they tempt the taste buds, make food more enjoyable and give meals a kick.

- Add fresh herbs – a few torn basil leaves, or a sprinkle of chopped coriander add a zesty zing to any dish.

- Use a smaller plate than normal – it kids your brain into thinking you're eating more!

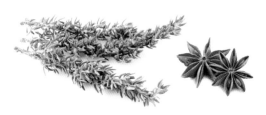

Make an occasion

Just because you're only eating 500 calories on two days of the week doesn't mean you should scoff standing up.

Make an occasion of every mouthful. Set the table with proper place mats. Pour a long cool glass of water and add a slice of lemon or lime for a zesty kick. Use proper linen napkins. Turn off the radio or television and make eating a real event. One of the reasons that many of us gain weight in the first place is that we eat without really noticing what we're putting into our mouths.

Use your fast days to really get reacquainted with food. Savour the texture, the taste, admire the wonderful hues on your plate and really enjoy them.

Eating with others

It certainly demands more willpower if you are eating with others on your fast days. You need a couple of weapons in your armoury – be firm if they try and tempt you, and explain calmly how much better you're feeling as a result of your 5:2 plan.

If you find it really hard to stay focused, especially if you're cooking for others, you might like to eat your own meal first. This allows you peace and quiet to concentrate and it also stops you picking and tasting as you cook. And it's only for a couple of days of the week – that very fact means that people around you are likely to be much more tolerant of your fast days.

Seasonal changes

We all change what we eat depending on the weather so let the seasons be your guide when it comes to the 5:2 diet. If it's warm outside, opt for plenty of fresh, wholesome salads and long, cool drinks. Eat al fresco if you can – being out in the sunshine works wonders for your moods. If it's chilly, steam cabbage and broccoli to add to your plate, or make hearty soups using low-calorie tinned tomatoes and passata as your base.

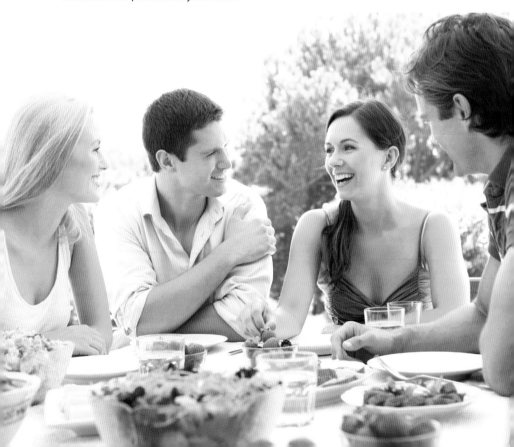

Motivation and Goal Setting

What's your motivation?

Any actress will tell you that in order to understand the character they are playing, they need to know why she's doing what she's doing. In other words, what's her motivation? The same goes for anyone on the 5:2 diet.

You need to know why you're doing it – and what you aim to get out of it. Research shows that people who have a clear goal in life are generally more likely to succeed. In other words, if you have a clear idea of exactly what you want, you're more likely to achieve it.

So, before you start this new way of eating, take a little time to consider why you're going on the 5:2 diet and what your goals are.

Most of us have both long and short-term goals. It's a good idea to have something close to aim for as well as something much further away. It means that you always have something new to work towards.

Short term

Short-term goals can be anything you like.

For example, you may want to shed a few pounds simply to get back into your jeans, or to get back to your usual weight after a particularly indulgent holiday. You may have a big event on the horizon, a wedding or birthday bash – and you don't want to feel like a lumpy frump. Maybe you've decided that all this extra weight isn't good for your health and you want to get yourself in shape? You could even be combining the 5:2 diet with a training plan for a fun run, or even a half marathon.

Don't consign resolutions to the New Year.
Plans for a new you can start any time!

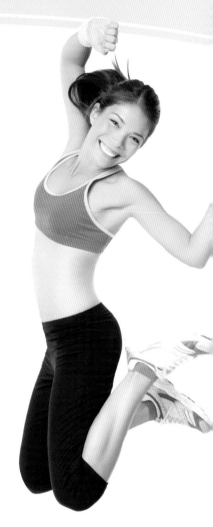

Long term

Just as it sounds, long-term goals are over-arching – they span a longer period and take more time to achieve. For you, it could be that you want weight loss to be part of a whole new life plan, a new direction you see yourself going in. Maybe you plan a career change in a few month's time and want to feel more confident about the way you look.

Perhaps you want to increase your overall health and know that being at the right weight for your height is all part of the process.

Take time

Whatever your aims, give yourself time and patience to get there. And with determination you'll succeed!

Reward yourself

Everyone likes a little pat on the back, and when you're trying to lose weight, it's even more important that you tell yourself 'well done' as you head towards your goal.

It doesn't have to be a big gesture; it needn't even cost much money. But do remember to treat yourself every time you reach a milestone. Whether you want to lose five pounds or five stone, take baby steps and reward yourself along the way.

Try some of these:

• A star chart. It works wonders for children, why not try it for yourself? Every time you lose a pound, give yourself a sticker. Then say, when you lose five pounds, you can 'cash' that in for a little low-cost reward, a new magazine, or a jazzy pair of socks. Silly socks can be a great motivator – as while you're waiting to slip into the next size jeans, feet tend to stay the same size. The rough guide is that for every 15 pounds you lose, you also go down a dress size, so you'll only have to 'earn' yourself three pairs of jazzy socks before those jeans fit!

• A pebble jar. Get an empty jar, and every time you lose a pound, put a pebble in it. Watch the jar fill up as you lose weight.

• A weight bag. Get yourself a 'bag for life' and every time you lose a pound, find a household item that weighs roughly the same. You'll be amazed just how much weight you've lost every time you pick up the bag. And think how much more energetic you'll feel without those extra pounds hanging on to your hips!

- Chart it! Draw yourself a graph and map your progress. This can be really useful on difficult weeks. If you see the graph spike upwards, it can give you the motivation to focus and get that line heading south.

- Save it! On your fast days, as you're only going to be eating 500 calories, there's a good chance you'll be saving money. Work out what your usual daily menus would have cost and pop the coins you've saved in a special piggy bank. At the end of the diet, tip them out and treat yourself.

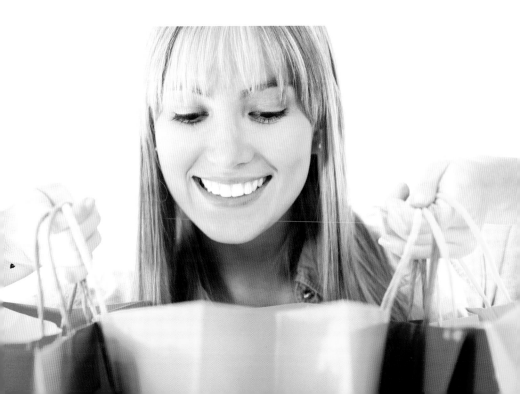

Being Active

Now is the time to get active. We're constantly being told that we're a nation of couch potatoes so it's wise to incorporate exercise into all areas of your life. Our sedentary lives, working at computers and watching television, can lead to weight gain. And once we've got used to sitting around so much, it can be hard to push ourselves to get moving.

If catching up with the soaps, or sitting down with a good book, is one of your preferred pastimes, don't worry. You don't have to give it up. Instead, it's a good idea to try and incorporate exercise into your daily life.

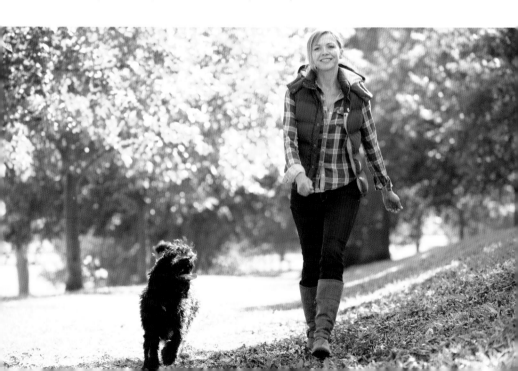

If that thought makes you groan, don't despair. If you're one of those people who hated gym lessons as a kid, it's not the end of the world. You don't have to rush out and take up a sport you loathe.

It's all about keeping moving and making activity an integral part of every day. Start simply – walk about while you talk on the phone, get up and do a few stretches every 20 minutes or so if you're tied to a computer during your working day. If you take usually take the lift, then choose the stairs instead. It might seem tough to begin with, but it will get easier every day.

Why exercise?

Making the effort to keep active every day helps keep your heart healthy, reduces your risk of serious illness and strengthens muscles and bones.

It can help give you better results while you're dieting too – helping your weight loss and toning up muscles as well. It also means you're more likely to keep to your desired weight even after you stop doing the 5:2 diet.

If you're new to regular exercise or have any specific health conditions, do ensure you consult your GP first before taking up any kind of fitness regime.

Timetable it

You don't have to set certain times aside for exercise, just add it in to your everyday timetable. For example, if you get the bus to work, get off two or three stops earlier and walk the rest of the way. If you're going shopping, park the car at the very far end of the supermarket. Do you normally just nip the dog round the block? Then make time for a longer walk. Post those letters at another post box rather than the one on the corner.

Fit it in

Make ordinary chores more energetic. Not only will you get better results around the house, you'll start to feel fitter too. Really put some elbow grease into cleaning those windows, be really vigorous when you're mopping the kitchen floor. Pop some high-energy music on when you're hovering – not only will it boost your mood, you'll find you move more too.

On the cheap

There are plenty of ways to boost your activity levels without spending much at all (if anything).

Try this:

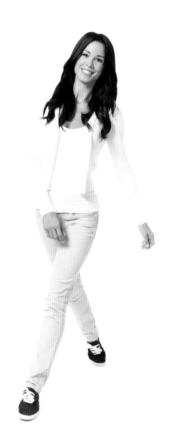

• The great outdoors is just beyond the door. Step out and gradually build up your speed and the distance you go each day. It doesn't matter whether you live in a town or a tiny village – there are plenty of places to walk. Get more acquainted with your locality. Even if you live in an inner city, take time to stride out. You'll be amazed how good it makes you feel. And you'll spot all kinds of things you miss when you're driving – urban architecture, interesting shops, pretty plants and beautiful birds.

- Borrow a dog. If you haven't got one, there's bound to be a friend or neighbour who's happy to lend you Rover for an extra walk.

- If you have children, get them walking with you. They might moan to start with but offer them non-food incentives. By taking them with you you're setting a fantastic example.

- Swimming. Most local leisure centres offer low-cost swim times. Swimming is a great form of exercise, whatever your shape. Because it's non-weight bearing, it places less pressure on the joints – and it gives you a wonderful feeling of weightlessness. Swimming is great at any time of day but fabulous first thing as it sets you up for the day. An evening swim is worth a look too and can lead to a great night's sleep.

- Dance away. Pop on the radio or your MP3 and off you go. Dance round the kitchen, hula hula through the hall and waltz around the living room. Again, dance is one of those activities which is good for your mood as well as your body!

- Wash the car. Not just a cursory wipe. Get a big bucket full of car shampoo and scrub away. The benefit means you have a super sparkly vehicle and you're burning calories too.

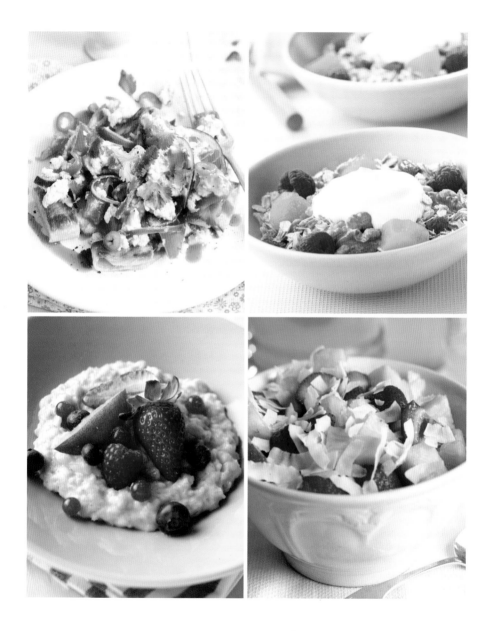

Breakfast

Breakfast is exactly that, the original breaking of the fast. If you ate your last meal over 12 hours ago, you're probably going to want to include a breakfast option on your fast days.

Taking breakfast has certain advantages in that it peps up your metabolism and gives you energy for your day ahead. If you want to make the most of your calories, start the day with a glass of water with a squeeze of lemon. Not only does this provide essential hydration, it also stops you craving too many calories.

Healthy Mexican Eggs

Serves: **2** | Preparation time: **5 minutes**
Cooking time: **10 minutes** | Calories per portion: **284**

Ingredients

- 1 tbsp olive oil
- ½ red onion, sliced
- 2 medium tomatoes, cubed
- 1 Jalapeno chilli (chili), sliced
- 1 flour tortilla
- 3 large eggs, lightly beaten
- 2 tbsp sweet chilli (chili) sauce
- 1 tbsp coriander (cilantro) leaves, roughly chopped

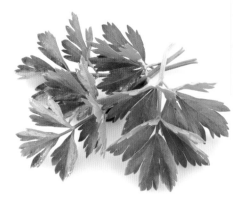

Method

1. Heat the oil in a frying pan and fry the onion for 2 minutes to soften. Add the tomatoes and chilli and warm through for 1 minute. Remove from the pan with a slotted spoon and keep warm.

2. Put the pan back over a high heat and cook the tortilla for 2 minutes on each side or until golden brown. Roll up the tortilla and cut it across into thick ribbons, then divide between two warm plates.

3. Put the pan back over a low heat, then pour in the eggs. Stir constantly until they scramble, then stir in the onion mixture.

4. Spoon the eggs over the tortilla ribbons and drizzle with sweet chilli sauce. Sprinkle with coriander and serve immediately.

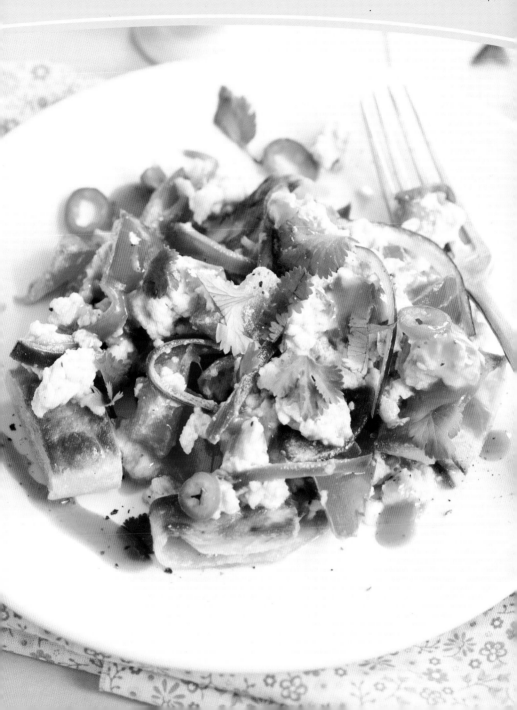

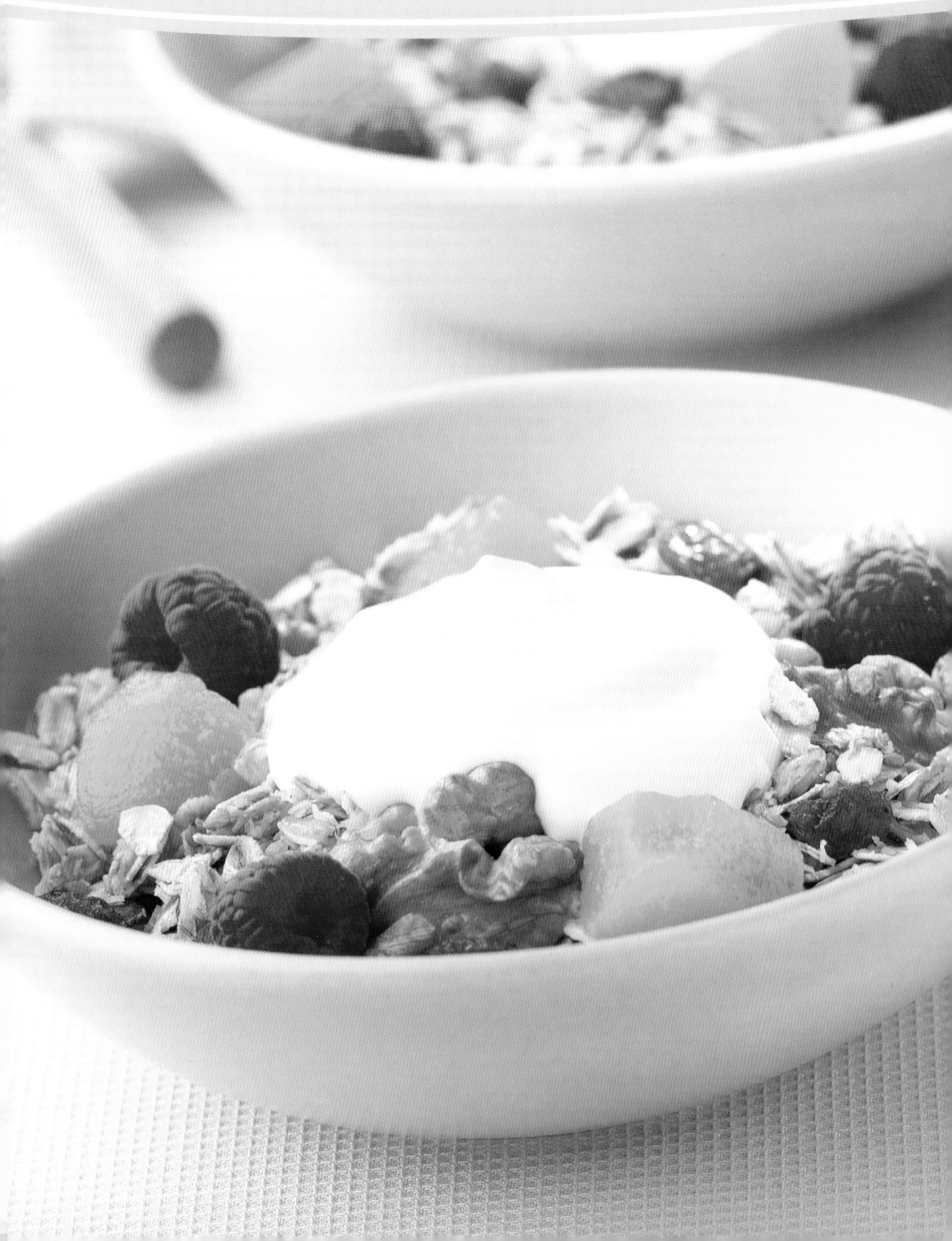

Fruity Yoghurt Muesli

Serves: **2** | Preparation time: **5 minutes**
Calories per portion: **315**

Ingredients

- 100 g / 3 ½ oz / 1 cup jumbo porridge oats
- 2 tbsp desiccated coconut
- 6 walnut halves
- 2 tbsp sultanas
- 50 g / 1 ¾ oz / ¼ cup 0% fat Greek yoghurt
- ½ ripe peach, skinned and stoned
- 6 raspberries

Method

1. Mix the oats with the coconut and divide between 2 bowls.

2. Share out the walnut halves and sultanas, then spoon over the yoghurt.

3. Chop the peach into bite-sized chunks and divide between the 2 bowls with the raspberries.

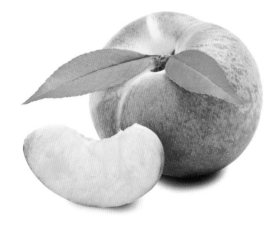

Summer Fruit Porridge

Serves: **1** | Preparation time: **5 minutes**
Cooking time: **7 minutes** | Calories per portion: **227**

Ingredients

- 40 g / 1 ½ oz / ½ cup oatmeal
- ½ tsp vanilla extract
- 2 tsp runny honey
- 50 g / 1 ½ oz / ⅓ cup mixed summer fruit

Method

1. Boil 150 ml of water in a saucepan, then stir in the oatmeal and a pinch of salt.

2. Simmer the porridge over a low heat for 5–6 minutes, stirring occasionally. Add a little more water if it gets too thick.

3. Turn off the heat, cover the pan and leave the porridge to stand for 1 minute.

4. Stir in the vanilla extract and honey, then spoon the porridge into a bowl and top with the fruit.

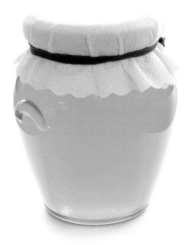

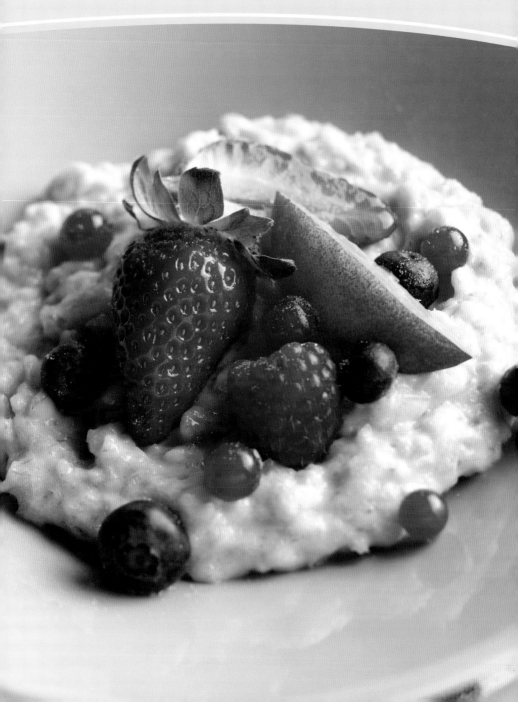

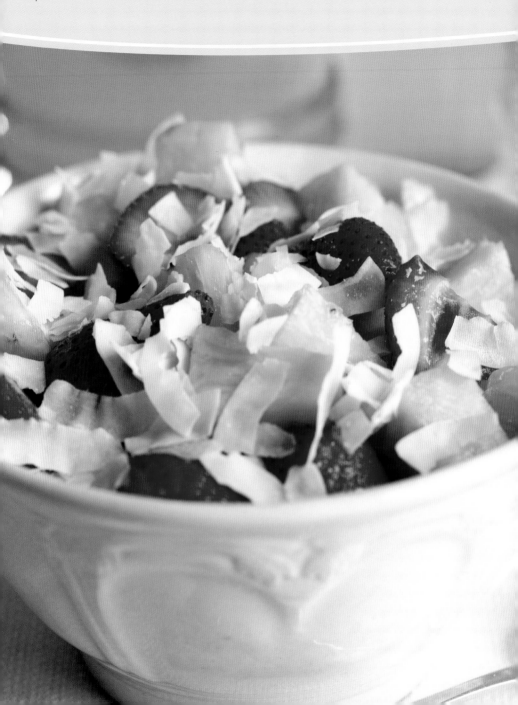

Coconut Fruit Salad

Serves: **4** | Preparation time: **10 minutes**
Calories per portion: **134**

Ingredients

- 1 medium pineapple, peeled and cored
- 400 g / 14 oz / 2 ⅔ cups strawberries, halved
- 28 g / 1 oz / ⅓ cup unsweetened dried coconut flakes

Method

1. Cut the pineapple into 8 wedges, then cut each wedge across into bite-sized chunks.

2. Mix the pineapple with the strawberry halves, then divide between 4 bowls.

3. Sprinkle over the coconut flakes and serve immediately.

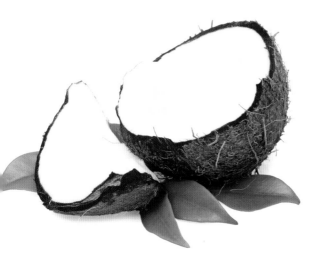

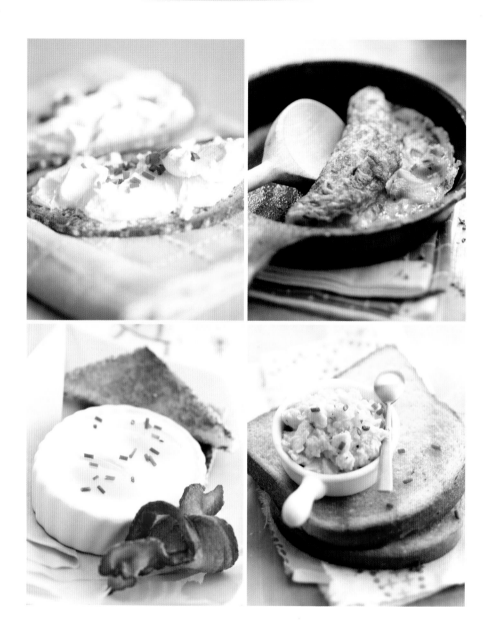

Brunch

If you're one of those people who's never hungry first thing, then brunch might be perfect for you. The term 'brunch' was originally coined by Punch magazine in 1896 as a term used for a meal taken late Sunday mornings by people who'd been out on the town.

Brunch can be whatever you want – a cross between breakfast and lunch. It can be a great meal to have as part of your fast day calories, as it means you 'save' by not having breakfast.

Cream Cheese On Rye

Serves: **2** | Preparation time: **2 minutes**
Calories per portion: **256**

Ingredients

- 4 thin slices rye bread
- 125 g / 4 ½ oz / ½ cup low fat soft cheese
- 1 tbsp fresh chives, chopped

Method

1. Spread the bread with the cheese and sprinkle with the chopped chives.

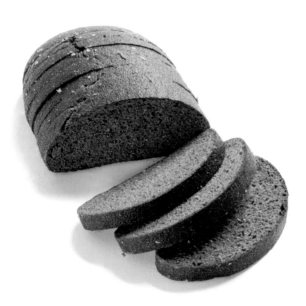

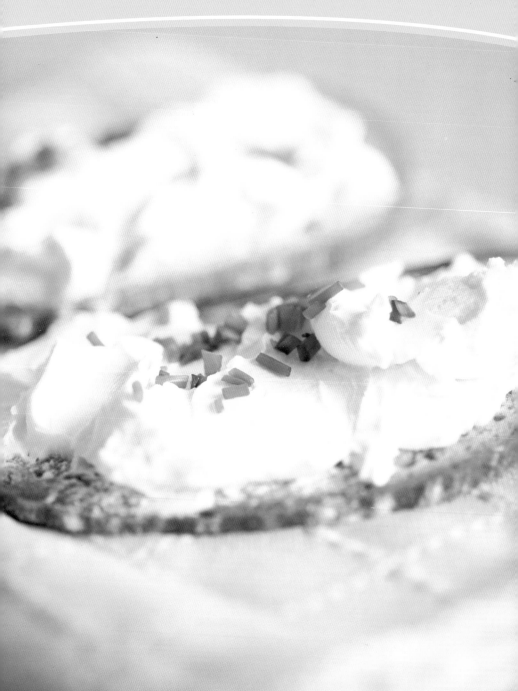

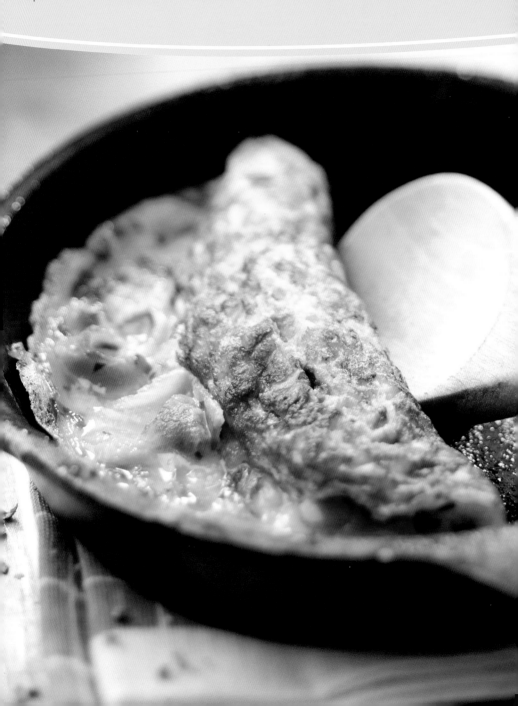

Herby Bacon Omelette

Serves: **1** | Preparation time: **2 minutes**
Cooking time: **6 minutes** | Calories per portion: **219**

Ingredients

- 1 rasher unsmoked back bacon, chopped
- 2 large eggs
- 2 tbsp flat leaf parsley, chopped

Method

1. Fry the bacon in a dry frying pan for 2 minutes to release some of the fat, then remove it from the pan with a slotted spoon and reserve.
2. Lightly beat the eggs with the parsley and a pinch of salt and pepper.
3. Pour the mixture into the frying pan and cook over a medium heat until it starts to set around the outside.
4. Use a spatula to draw the sides of the omelette into the centre then tilt the pan to fill the gaps with more liquid egg.
5. Repeat the process until the top of the omelette is almost set then sprinkle over the bacon pieces.
6. Fold the omelette in half and serve immediately.

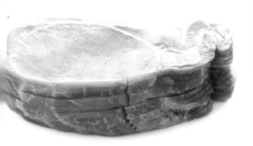

Coddled Eggs

Serves: **1** | Preparation time: **2 minutes**
Cooking time: **6–8 minutes** | Calories per portion: **145**

Ingredients

- 4 sprays of 1-cal sunflower oil spray
- 2 large eggs
- ½ tsp fresh chives, chopped

Method

1. Spray a ramekin dish with oil, then break in the eggs.

2. Place the dish in a saucepan and pour enough boiling water around the outside of the dish to come half way up the sides.

3. Put a lid on the pan and simmer gently for 6–8 minutes or until the egg white has set, but the yolks are still runny.

4. Carefully remove the eggs from the ramekin and sprinkle with chives before serving.

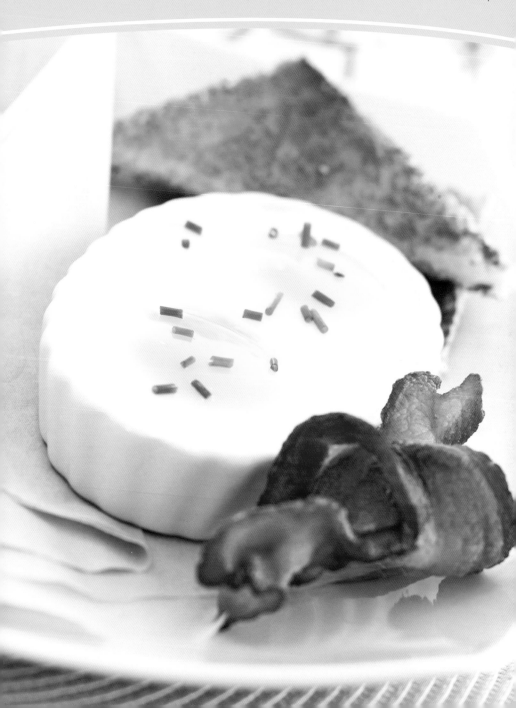

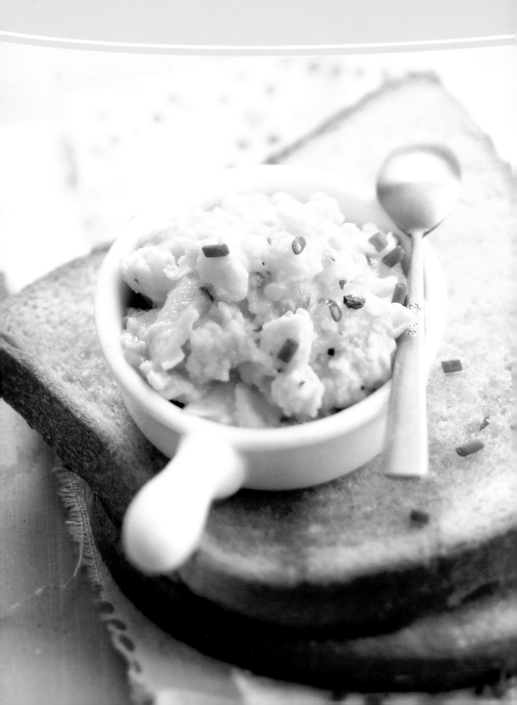

Scrambled Egg On Toast

Serves: **1** | Preparation time: **2 minutes**

Cooking time: **4 minutes** | Calories per portion: **238**

Ingredients

- 2 slices reduced calorie white bread
- 2 large eggs
- 1 tsp fresh chives, chopped
- a pinch of ground pink peppercorns

Method

1. Toast the bread and keep it warm while you make the scramble.

2. Break the eggs into a small saucepan and beat them gently with a pinch of salt.

3. Turn on the heat under the pan and stir the eggs until they scramble, then spoon them into a small bowl.

4. Sprinkle the top with the chives and pink pepper, then serve immediately with the toast.

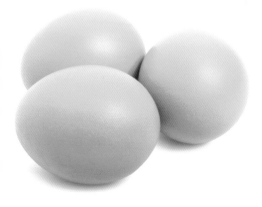

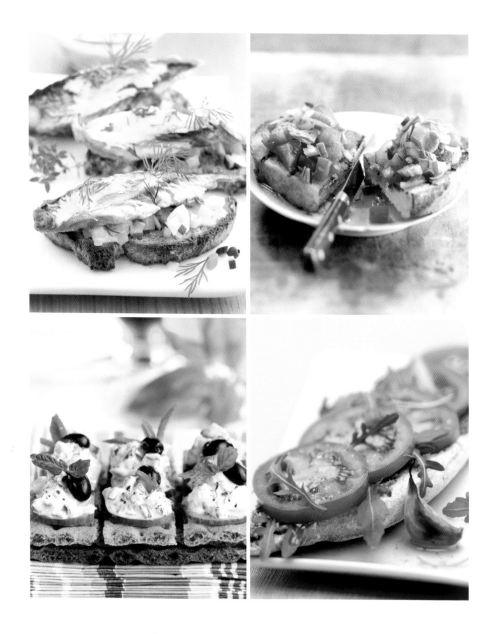

Light Lunches

These lunch ideas can actually be eaten at other times of the day and would work equally well as dinners. Several of them are easily portable too, for when you're at work or out and about.

We've put together a tasty selection of light lunches – some that need little or no cooking and others that require a little more work. Mix and match these ideas and see which ones work best for you.

Mackerel Bruschetta

Serves: **4** | Preparation time: **5 minutes**
Cooking time: **10 minutes** | Calories per portion: **352**

Ingredients

- 4 slices wholemeal granary bread
- 1 medium carrot, peeled and diced
- 1 medium courgette (zucchini), diced
- 2 small turnips, peeled and diced
- 100 ml / 3 ½ fl. oz / ½ cup white wine vinegar
- 5 allspice berries
- 4 fresh mackerel fillets

For the dressing:
- 100 g / 3 ½ oz / ½ cup 0% fat Greek yoghurt
- 1 tsp Dijon mustard
- 2 tbsp dill fronds, roughly chopped

Method

1. Toast the bread and keep it warm while you prepare the rest of the dish.

2. Put the vegetables in a saucepan with the vinegar and enough cold water to cover them. Add the allspice berries and ½ tsp of salt then simmer the vegetables for 6 minutes or until just tender. Drain well and discard the allspice.

3. Meanwhile, cook the mackerel fillets under a hot grill for 2 minutes on each side or until just cooked through.

4. Divide the pickled vegetables between the toast slices.

5. Mix the yoghurt with the mustard and dill then spoon half of it over the vegetables.

6. Top the vegetables with the mackerel fillets and spoon over the rest of the dressing.

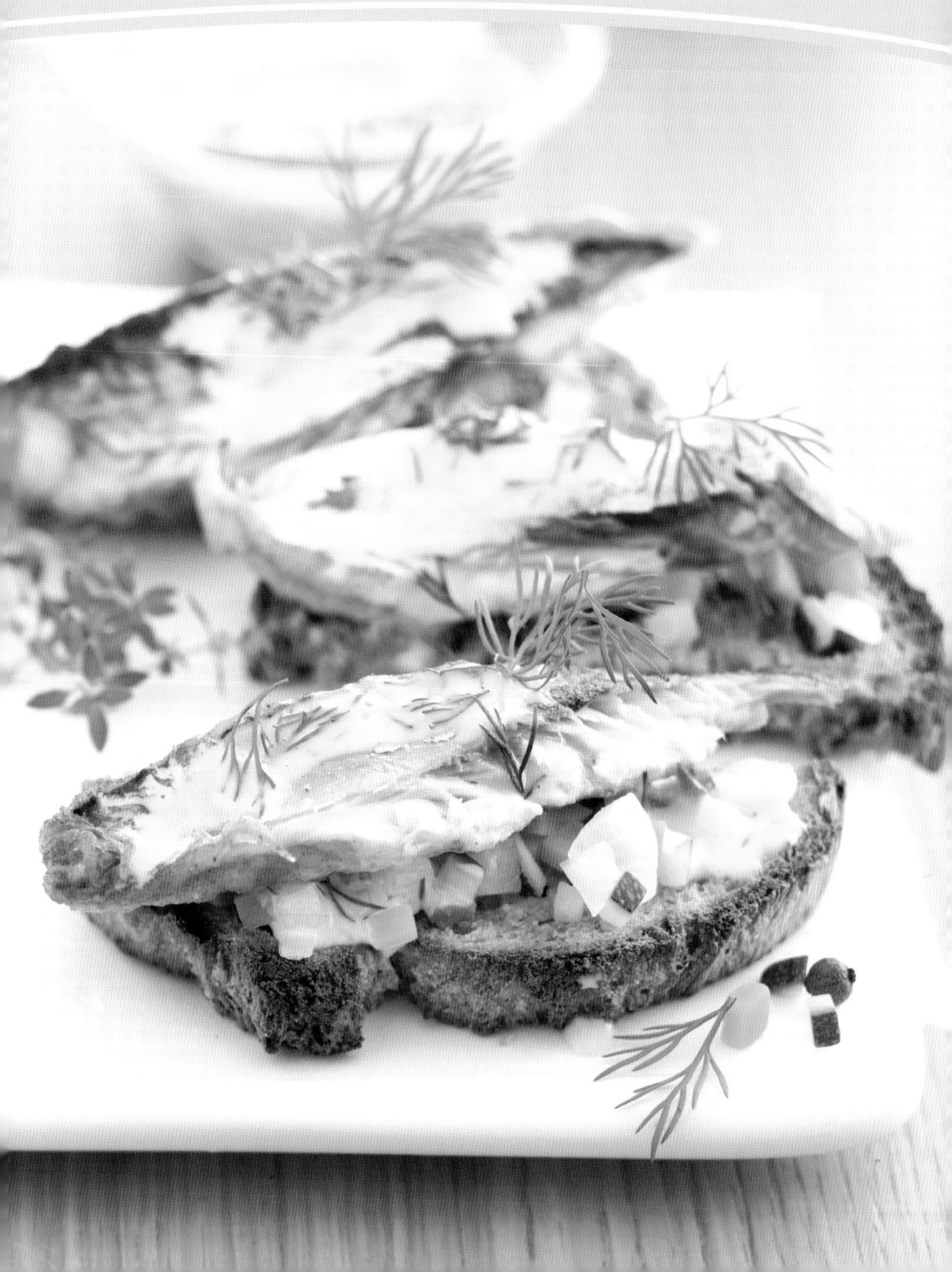

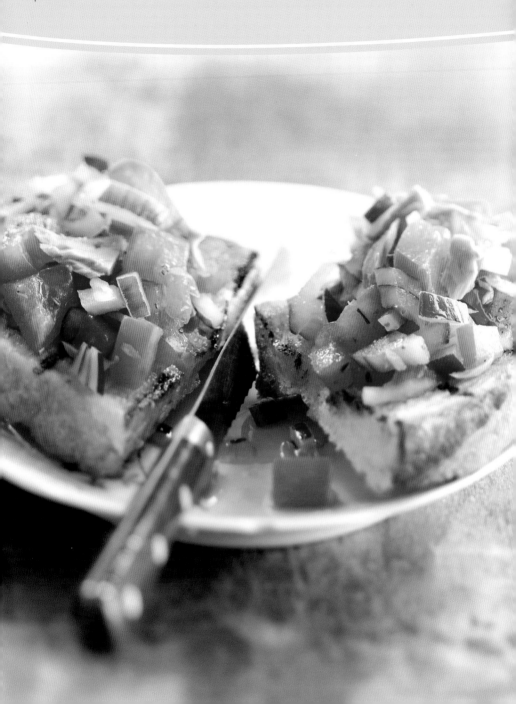

Tomato and Tuna Toasts

Serves: **2** | Preparation time: **5 minutes**

Cooking time: **4 minutes** | Calories per portion: **317**

Ingredients

- 185 g / 6 ½ oz can of tuna in spring water, drained
- 4 tomatoes, diced
- ½ red onion, diced
- a pinch of chopped parsley
- 2 tbsp extra virgin olive oil
- 2 slices reduced calorie white bread

Method

1. Flake the tuna into a bowl and mix it with the tomatoes, onion and parsley.

2. Stir in the oil and season to taste with salt and pepper.

3. Toast the bread in a hot griddle pan until nicely marked, then transfer it to 2 warm plates.

4. Top the toast with the tuna mixture and serve immediately.

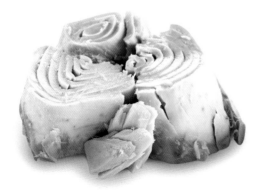

Tzatziki On Crispbread

Serves: **4** | Preparation time: **25 minutes**
Calories per portion: **127**

Ingredients

- 1 medium cucumber
- 100 g / 3 ½ oz / ½ cup 0% fat Greek yoghurt
- 1 clove of garlic, crushed
- 2 spring onions (scallions), finely chopped
- 2 tsp lemon juice
- 1 tbsp mint leaves, chopped, plus extra to garnish
- 8 rye crispbreads
- 16 black olives in brine, pitted
- freshly ground black pepper

Method

1. Cut 16 slices from the cucumber and set them aside. Cut the rest of the cucumber in half lengthways and scrape out the seeds with a teaspoon.
2. Finely chop the flesh and put it in a sieve, then sprinkle with salt and leave to drip for 15 minutes.
3. Mix the yoghurt with the garlic, spring onion, lemon juice and mint. Blot the cucumber flesh with kitchen paper, then fold it into the yoghurt dressing.
4. Arrange 2 cucumber slices on top of each crispbread, then add a spoonful of tzatziki to each.
5. Garnish with black olives, mint sprigs and a sprinkle of freshly ground black pepper. Serve two crispbreads per person.

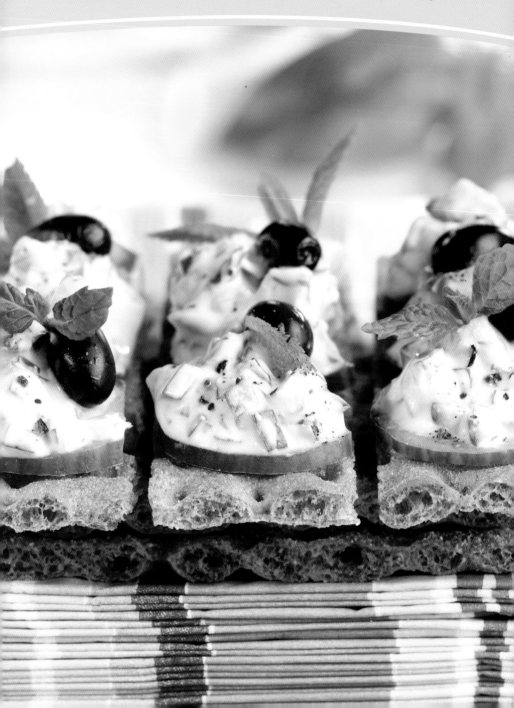

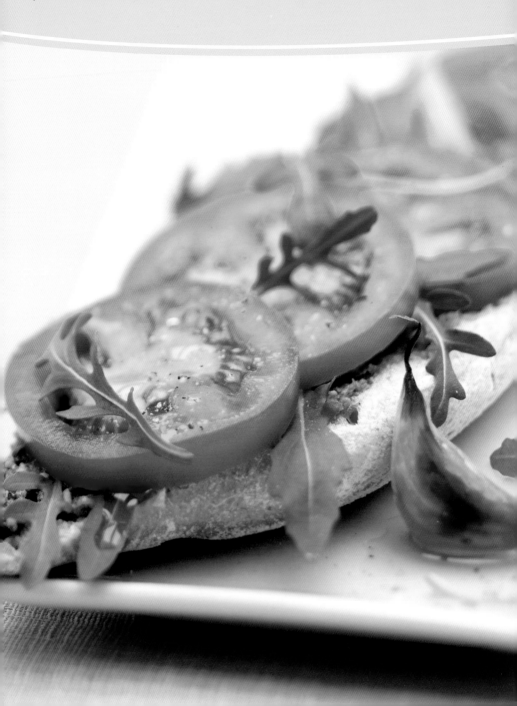

Tomato Bruschetta

Serves: **1** | Preparation time: **5 minutes**
Calories per portion: **216**

Ingredients

- ½ rustic bread roll
- 1 tbsp pesto
- 1 medium tomato, sliced
- a few rocket (arugula) leaves
- 1 tsp extra virgin olive oil
- salt and freshly ground black pepper

Method

1. Spread the bread roll with pesto and top with the tomato slices.

2. Scatter over the rocket leaves and drizzle with olive oil, then season with salt and pepper.

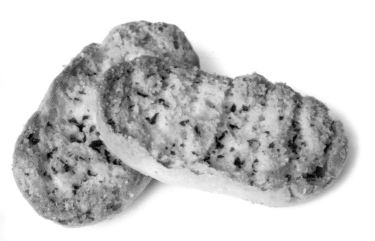

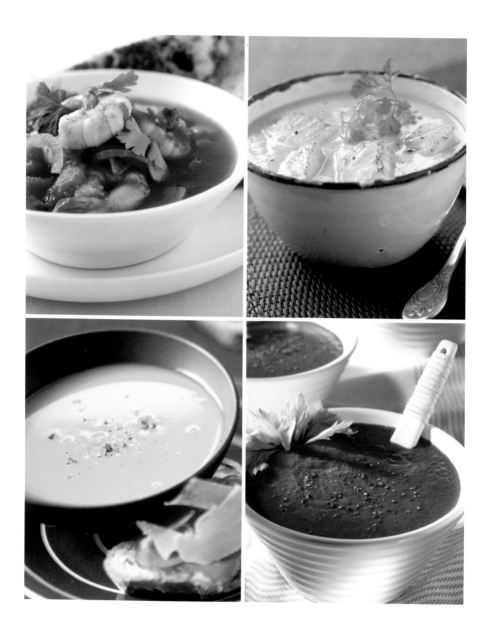

Soups

Soups make a nourishing, filling and warming addition to your fast day recipes. The wonderful thing about soup is that it makes you feel like you're getting a lot for a little. Using plenty of vegetables is also good news on many counts – you get lots of additional vitamins, minerals and fibre.

Ring the changes in how you serve soups. Choose a large mug for a huggably hot drink, or invest in pretty little mini soup tureens. Decorate your soups with fresh herbs for additional tones. Yum!

Prawn and Tomato Soup

Serves: **2** | Preparation time: **5 minutes**
Cooking time: **20 minutes** | Calories per portion: **251**

Ingredients

- 2 tsp olive oil
- 1 onion, quartered and sliced
- 3 cloves of garlic, crushed
- ½ tsp smoked paprika
- 1 tbsp concentrated tomato purée
- 400 g / 14 oz / 1 ⅔ cups canned tomatoes, chopped
- 800 ml / 1 pint 8 fl. oz / 3 ¼ cups vegetable or fish stock
- 250 g / 9 oz / 1 ⅔ cups raw king prawns, peeled
- a few sprigs of flat leaf parsley, roughly chopped
- salt and freshly ground black pepper

Method

1. Heat the olive oil in a saucepan, then fry the onion over a medium heat for 5 minutes or until translucent.

2. Add the garlic and fry for 2 more minutes, then stir in the paprika and tomato purée.

3. Add the chopped tomatoes and stock to the pan, then simmer for 8 minutes. Taste the soup and season with salt and black pepper.

4. Stir the king prawns into the soup, then simmer gently for 2 minutes or until they just turn opaque and start to curl up.

5. Serve the soup immediately, sprinkled with the parsley.

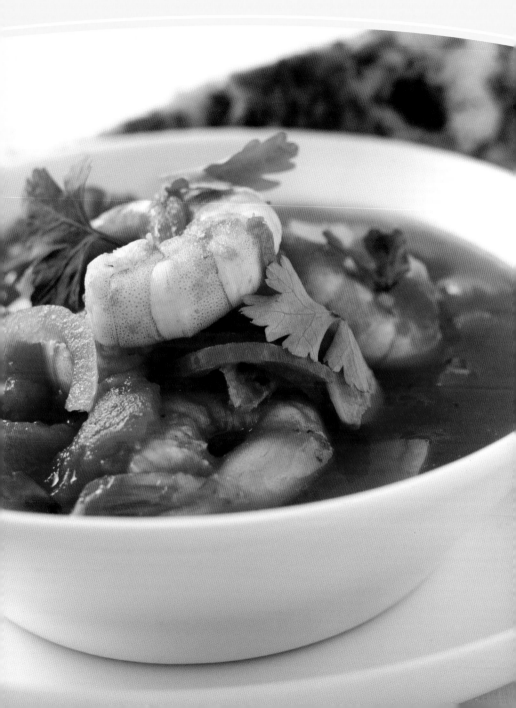

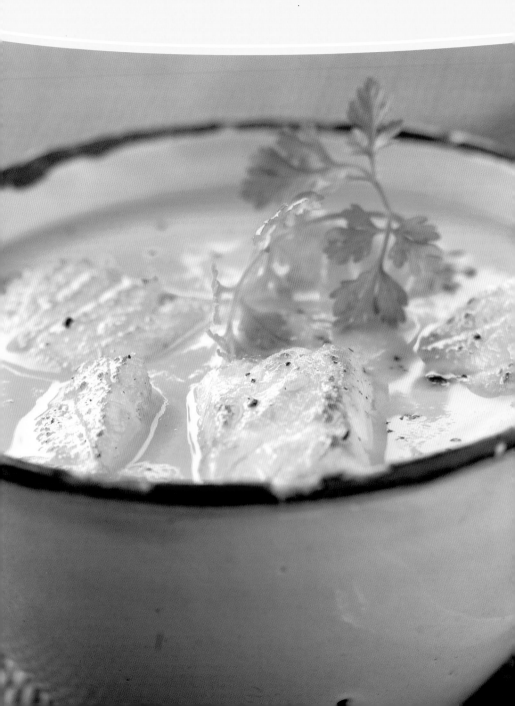

Carrot and Salmon Soup

Serves: **4** | Preparation time: **5 minutes**
Cooking time: **35–40 minutes** | Calories per portion: **165**

Ingredients

- ½ tsp caraway seeds
- ½ tsp coriander (cilantro) seeds
- 1 leek, diced
- 400 g / 14 oz / 1 ⅔ cups carrots, peeled and diced
- 1 ½ l / 2 ½ pt / 6 cups vegetable or fish stock
- 250 g / 9 oz salmon fillet, skinned
- a few sprigs of chervil
- salt and freshly ground black pepper

Method

1. Measure the caraway and coriander seeds into a large saucepan and dry-fry for 2 minutes or until lightly toasted and fragrant. Grind to a powder with a pestle and mortar.

2. Return the ground spices to the pan and add the leek, carrots and stock. Boil gently for 30 minutes or until the carrots are really tender.

3. Transfer the soup to a liquidiser and blend until smooth.

4. Return the soup to the saucepan and season to taste with salt and pepper.

5. Cut the salmon into bite-sized chunks and poach it gently in the soup over a low heat for 2 minutes or until it turns opaque.

6. Serve the soup garnished with fresh chervil.

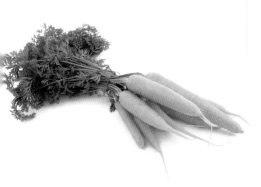

Spiced Pumpkin Soup

Serves: **4** | Preparation time: **5 minutes**
Cooking time: **35–40 minutes** | Calories per portion: **145**

Ingredients

- ½ tsp pink peppercorns, crushed
- ½ tsp cumin seeds
- ½ tsp chilli (chili) flakes
- 1 leek, diced
- 400 g / 14 oz / 1 ⅔ cups pumpkin, peeled and diced
- 1 ½ l / 2 ½ pt / 6 cups vegetable stock
- 4 slices reduced calorie white bread
- 4 thin slices Parma ham
- 20 g / ¾ oz aged Gouda
- salt and freshly ground black pepper

Method

1. Reserve half of the pink peppercorns for garnish and put the rest in a large saucepan with the cumin seeds and chilli flakes. Dry-fry for 2 minutes, then grind to a powder with a pestle and mortar.

2. Return the spices to the pan and add the leek, pumpkin and stock. Boil gently for 30 minutes or until the pumpkin is tender.

3. Transfer the soup to a liquidiser and blend until smooth. Season to taste with salt and pepper, then reheat gently.

4. Lightly toast the bread and top with the ham. Use a vegetable peeler to thinly slice the cheese over the top.

5. Ladle the soup into bowls and sprinkle with crushed pink peppercorns. Serve with the cheese and ham toasts.

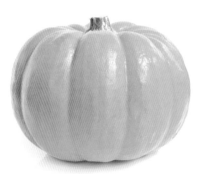

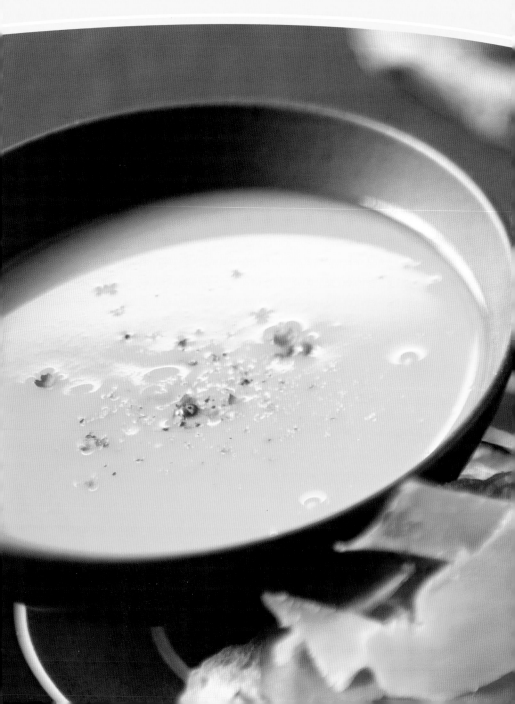

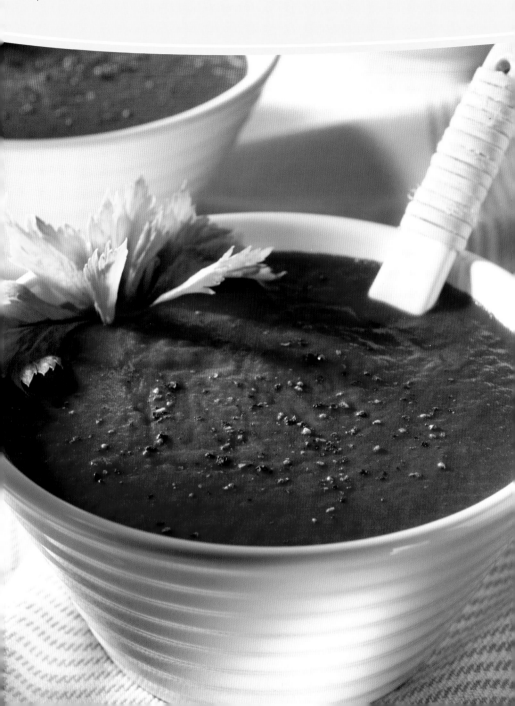

Beetroot and Celery Soup

Serves: **4** | Preparation time: **10 minutes**
Cooking time: **1 hour** | Calories per portion: **108**

Ingredients

- 1 tbsp olive oil
- 1 onion, finely chopped
- 1 medium carrot, finely chopped
- 4 celery sticks, chopped and leaves reserved
- 400 g / 14 oz / 1 ⅔ cups beetroot, peeled and diced
- 1 ½ l / 2 ½ pt / 6 cups vegetable stock
- 1 tsp celery salt
- 1 salt and freshly ground black pepper

Method

1. Heat the oil in a large saucepan, then fry the onion for 5 minutes or until softened. Add the carrot and celery and sweat over a low heat for 10 minutes.

2. Add the beetroot, stock and celery salt to the pan then boil for 40 minutes or until the beetroot is tender.

3. Transfer the soup to a liquidiser and blend until smooth. Season to taste with salt and pepper, then serve garnished with celery leaves and black pepper.

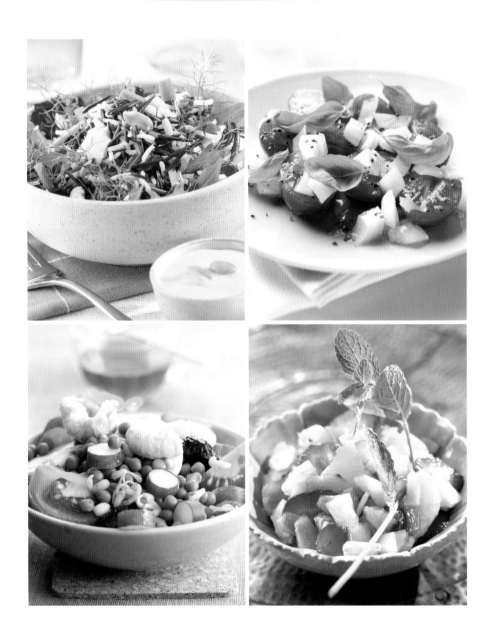

Salads

These days there is a wonderful and fresh array of salad vegetables available in almost every supermarket. Sometimes, there's even too much to choose from. Salads can be your best friend on fast days. They are very low in calories and also have the added advantage that they can take a lot of time to eat.

Make your salad choices as varied as possible to ensure you get the best mix of vitamins and minerals. Choose ruby red peppers, glossy cucumbers, crisp white onions and a razzmatazz of rocket and tomatoes. Salads make great portable lunches too, for when you're on the move.

Wild Rice Salad

Serves: **4** | Preparation time: **20 minutes**
Cooking time: **25 minutes** | Calories per portion: **204**

Ingredients

- 125 g / 4 ½ oz / ⅔ cup wild and long-grain rice, rinsed
- 1 medium carrot, peeled
- 1 radicchio lettuce
- 50 g / 1 ¾ oz / ½ cup rocket (arugula) leaves
- 2 tbsp raw peanuts
- a few sprigs of dill

For the dressing:

- 1 tbsp lime juice
- 1 tbsp smooth peanut butter
- 2 tbsp light mayonnaise

Method

1. Put the rice in a saucepan with 250 ml cold water. When the water starts to boil, cover the pan and turn the heat right down, then simmer for 20 minutes.

2. Turn off the heat, cover and leave to stand for 10 minutes. Fluff up the grains with a fork and leave to cool to room temperature.

3. While the rice is cooling, cut the carrot into matchsticks and slice the radicchio lettuce into ribbons.

4. For the dressing, stir the lime juice into the peanut butter to make a smooth paste, then stir in the mayonnaise.

5. Toss the rice with the carrots, radicchio, rocket, peanuts and dill. Divide between four bowls and serve alongside the dressing.

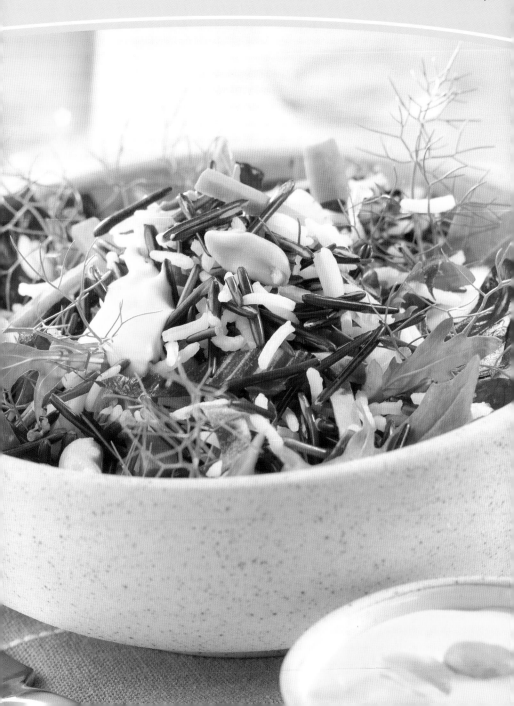

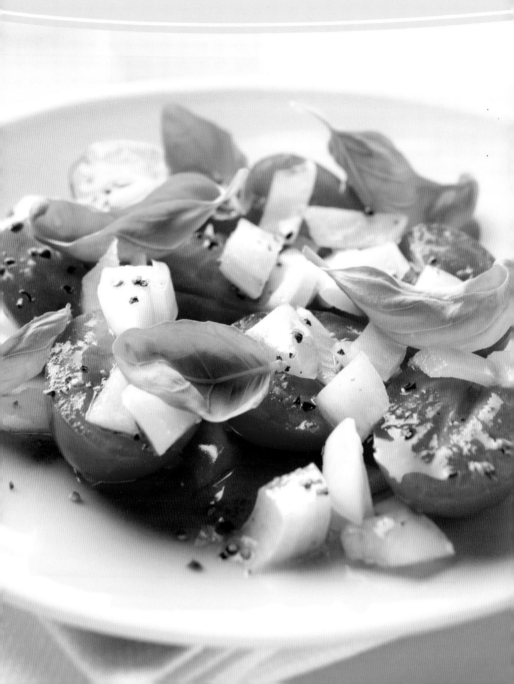

Tomato and Onion Salad

Serves: **2** | Preparation time: **5 minutes**
Calories per portion: **102**

Ingredients

- 350 g / 12 oz / 2 cups small tomatoes
- ½ white onion, diced
- freshly ground black pepper
- 1 tbsp extra virgin olive oil
- a handful of fresh basil leaves

Method

1. Slice the tomatoes in half and arrange them on two plates.

2. Scatter over the onion then sprinkle with freshly ground black pepper and drizzle with olive oil.

3. Garnish with fresh basil leaves.

Langoustine Salad

Serves: **4** | Preparation time: **5 minutes**

Cooking time: **4 minutes** | Calories per portion: **147**

Ingredients

- 300 g / 10 ½ oz / 2 cups frozen peas
- 400 g / 14 oz can of beansprouts, drained
- 2 tomatoes, sliced into wedges
- 100 g / 3 ½ oz / ¾ cup radishes, thickly sliced
- 12 black olives in oil, drained
- 100 g / 3 ½ oz / 1 cup cooked langoustine tails, peeled

Method

1. Boil the peas in salted water for 4 minutes, then drain and plunge into cold water. Drain well.

2. Toss the peas with the beansprouts, tomatoes and radishes and divide between 4 bowls.

3. Garnish with the olives and langoustine tails and serve immediately.

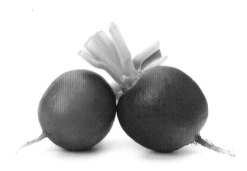

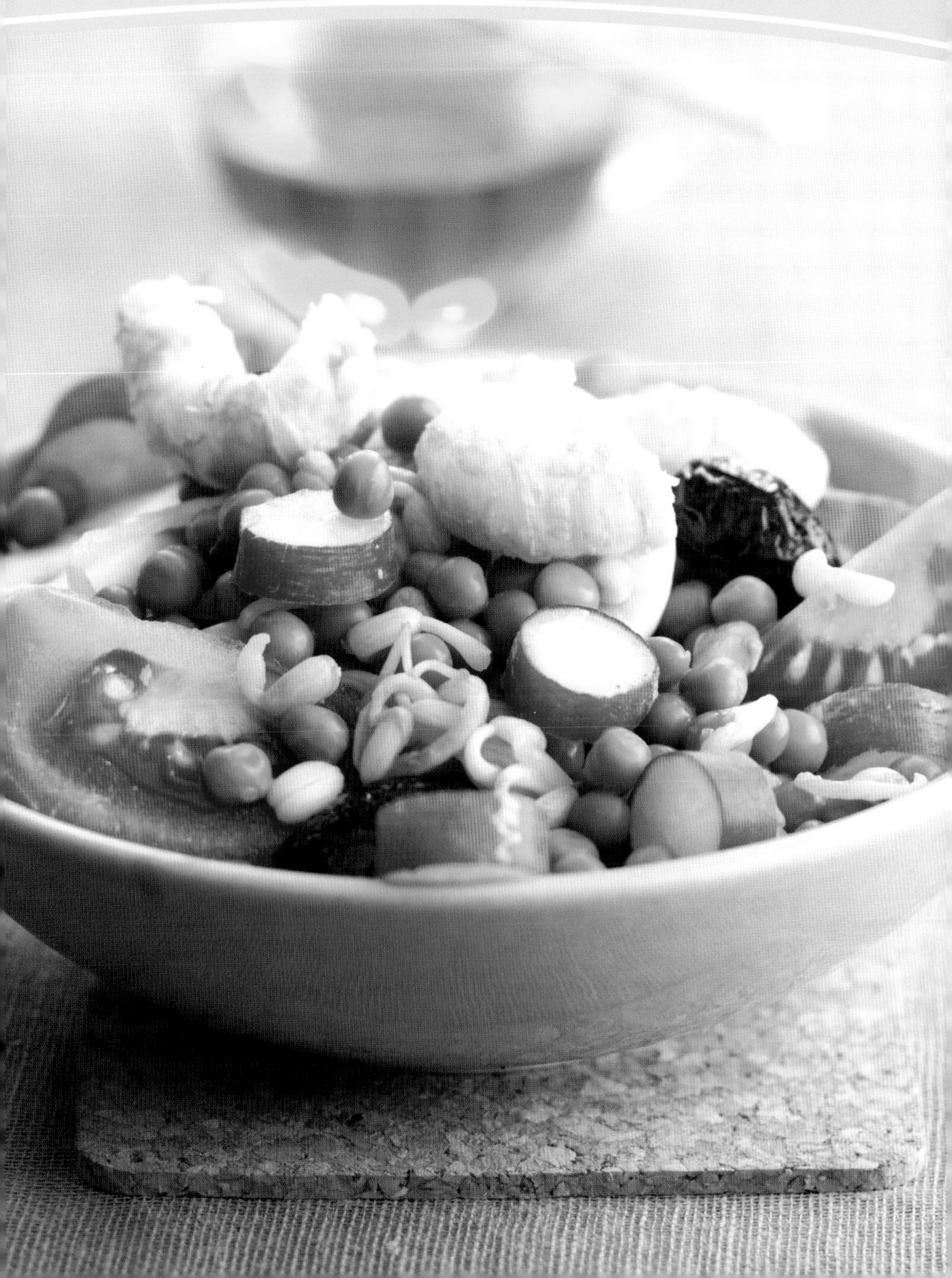

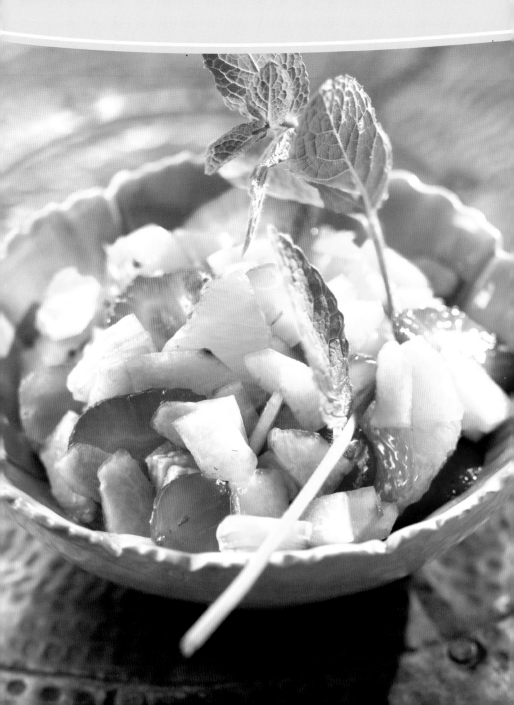

Cucumber Fruit Salad

Serves: **4** | Preparation time: **20 minutes**
Calories per portion: **81**

Ingredients

- 1 medium cucumber
- 1 navel orange
- 150 g / 5 ½ oz / 1 cup red seedless grapes
- 200 g / 7 oz / 1 ⅓ cups strawberries
- 2 tsp runny honey
- 2 limes, juiced
- 4 sprigs of mint

Method

1. Peel the cucumber and cut it lengthways into quarters, then cut it across into thin slices.

2. Use a sharp knife to slice the peel away from the orange, then cut out each individual segment.

3. Halve the grapes and slice the strawberries, then mix them together with the orange and cucumber in a bowl.

4. Dissolve the honey in the lime juice and pour it over the salad, then tuck in the mint sprigs and leave to marinate for 30 minutes before serving.

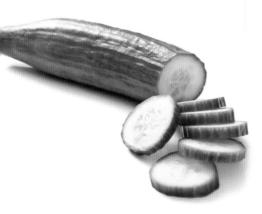

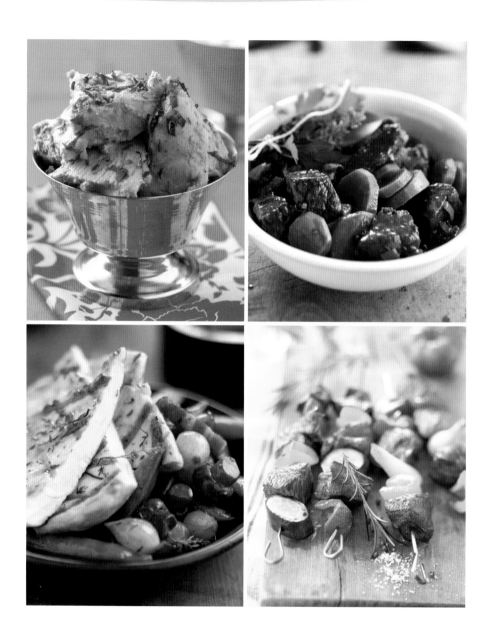

Meat

A range of meat fits perfectly well into the 5:2 diet so long as you stick to certain guidelines. Ensure you buy the leanest cuts of meat possible and remove all visible fat. If you're choosing poultry, always ensure that it is skinless as well. Many supermarkets offer a range of meats with different fat percentages so always choose the lowest fat content available.

Lean meat and poultry offer essential proteins, which are important on fast days. High protein foods can help you feel fuller for longer and also supply vital ingredients such as iron. A little protein can go a long way, so make sure you weigh everything carefully so you don't exceed your daily calorie limit.

Steamed Chicken Curry

Serves: **4** | Preparation time: **2 hours**

Cooking time: **8 minutes** | Calories per portion: **121**

Ingredients

- 400 g / 14 oz boneless skinless chicken breasts
- 50 g / 1 ¾ oz / ¼ cup 0% fat Greek yoghurt
- 1 tbsp curry powder
- ½ tsp dried chilli (chili) flakes
- 2 tbsp coriander (cilantro) leaves, chopped
- salt

Method

1. Cut the chicken breasts into large chunks and season with salt.

2. Mix the yoghurt with the curry powder and chilli flakes, then leave to marinate for 2 hours.

3. Transfer the chicken to a steamer basket and steam over a pan of boiling water for 8 minutes or until cooked through.

4. Divide between 4 warm bowls and serve sprinkled with coriander.

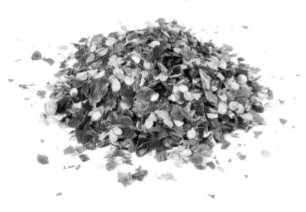

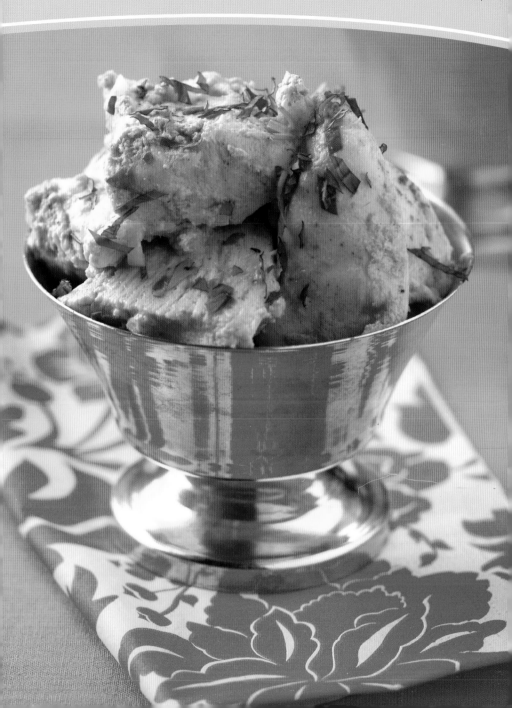

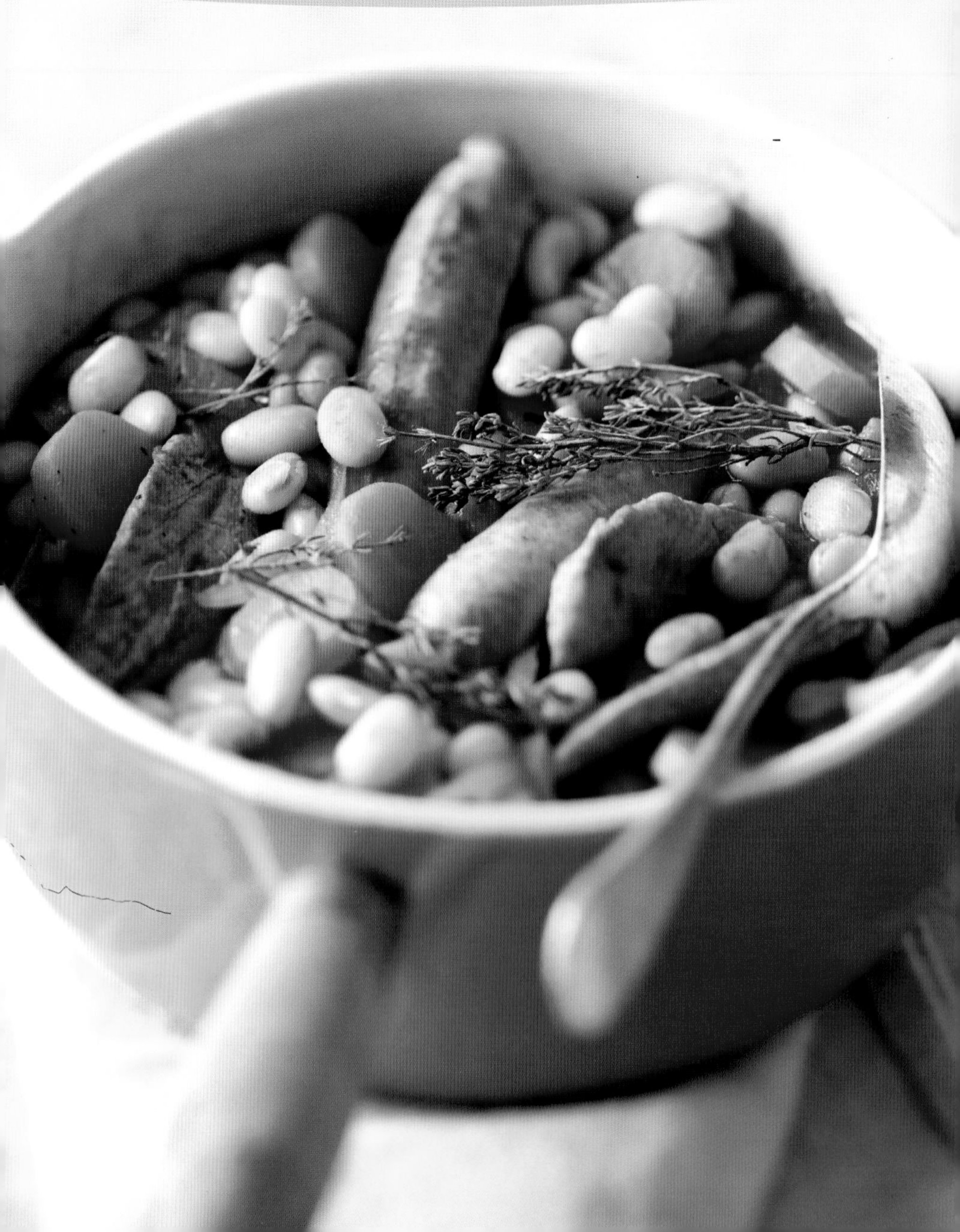

Pork and Bean Stew

Serves: **4** | Preparation time: **5 minutes**
Cooking time: **1 hour** | Calories per portion: **328**

Ingredients

- 1 tbsp olive oil
- 4 pork sausages
- 200 g / 7 oz lean pork escalope
- 1 onion, sliced
- 1 medium carrot, sliced
- 3 cloves of garlic, crushed
- 1 tbsp concentrated tomato purée
- 400 g / 14 oz can haricot beans, drained
- a few sprigs of thyme
- 450 ml / 16 fl. oz / 1 ¾ cups vegetable stock
- salt and freshly ground black pepper

Method

1. Heat the oil in a sauté pan, then brown the sausages and pork on all sides. Remove the meat from the pan and cut the pork into thick slices, then set aside.

2. Add the onion, carrot and garlic to the pan and sweat over a low heat for 10 minutes or until softened.

3. Stir in the tomato purée, haricot beans and thyme, then pour in the stock.

4. When the stock starts to boil, return the meat to the pan and reduce the heat. Simmer gently for 30 minutes, then season with salt and pepper before serving.

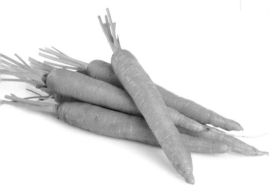

Chunky Chilli Con Carne

Serves: **4** | Preparation time: **5 minutes**
Cooking time: **45 minutes** | Calories per portion: **298**

Ingredients

- 400 g / 14 oz / 1 ¾ cups lean minced beef
- 1 tsp chilli (chili) powder
- 1 tsp dried oregano
- 450 ml / 16 fl. oz / 1 ¾ cups vegetable stock
- 250 g / 9 oz / 1 cup kidney beans
- 1 onion, sliced
- 4 cloves of garlic, unpeeled
- 250 g / 9 oz / 1 ⅔ cups tomatoes, cubed
- 1 tbsp olive oil
- a few sprigs of coriander (cilantro)
- salt and freshly ground black pepper

Method

1. Preheat the oven to 190°C (170°C fan) / 375F / gas 5.
2. Dry-fry the minced beef, chilli and oregano in a non-stick pan until browned.
3. Stir in the stock and kidney beans then simmer for 40 minutes or until tender.
4. Meanwhile, rub the onion, garlic and tomatoes with olive oil and spread out in a large roasting tin. Roast for 25 minutes, stirring occasionally.
5. Remove the garlic and set aside then stir the rest of the vegetables into the beef. Season to taste with salt and pepper, then divide the chilli con carne between four warm bowls.
6. Garnish each bowl with a roasted garlic clove and a sprig of coriander.

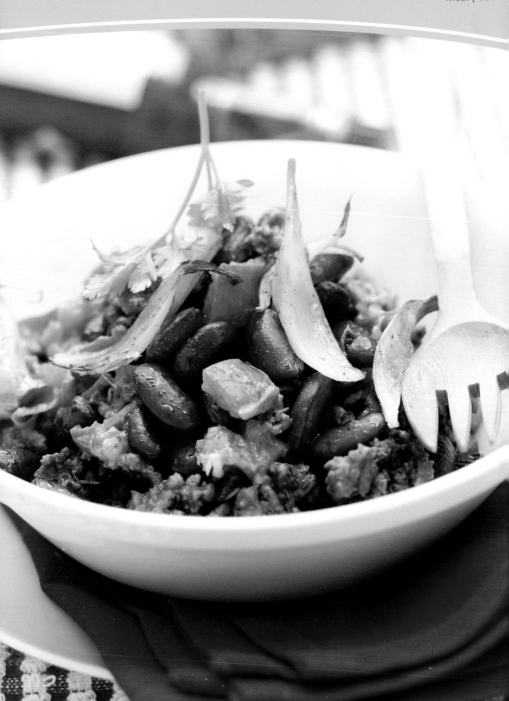

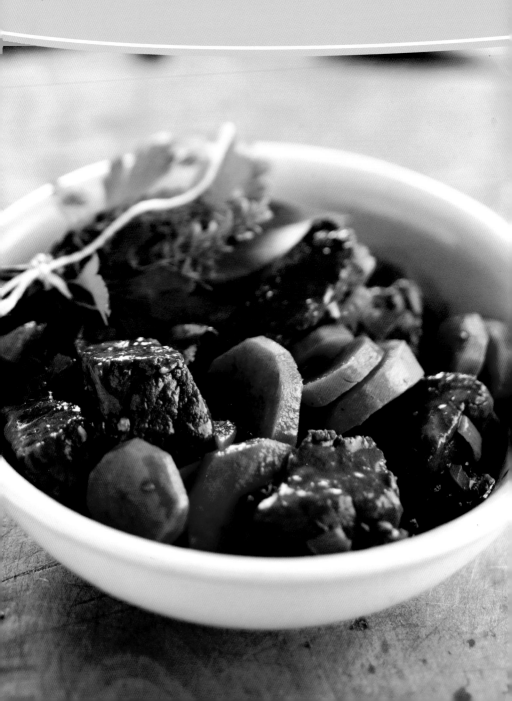

Beef and Carrot Stew

Serves: **4** | Preparation time: **5 minutes**
Cooking time: **2 hours 30 minutes** | Calories per portion: **367**

Ingredients

- 400 g / 14 oz / 1 ¾ cups lean braising steak, cubed
- 2 tbsp olive oil
- 1 onion, finely chopped
- 200 g / 7 oz / 1 ½ carrots, peeled and sliced
- 3 cloves of garlic, crushed
- 4 juniper berries, crushed
- 1 tbsp plain (all-purpose) flour
- 200 ml / 7 fl. oz / ¾ cup red wine
- 1 l / 1 pt 15 fl. oz / 4 cups beef stock
- 1 bouquet garni

Method

1. Dry the meat well with kitchen paper and season all over with salt and pepper.

2. Heat the oil in a large saucepan and brown the meat all over. Remove from the pan with a slotted spoon.

3. Add the onion, carrots, garlic and juniper berries and sweat over a low heat for 10 minutes to soften. Stir in the flour.

4. Increase the heat then pour in the wine and bubble away until almost evaporated.

5. Pour in the stock and add the bouquet garni. When the stock starts to boil, return the meat to the pan and reduce the heat. Simmer very gently for 2 hours or until the beef is tender.

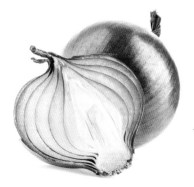

Turkey and Vegetables

Serves: **2** | Preparation time: **5 minutes**
Cooking time: **25 minutes** | Calories per portion: **346**

Ingredients

- 200 g / 7 oz turkey breast escalopes
- 2 tbsp olive oil
- 1 tbsp fresh thyme leaves
- 50 g / 1 ¾ oz / ½ cup smoked bacon lardons
- 100 g / 3 ½ oz / 1 cup pickling onions, peeled
- 100 g / 3 ½ oz / 1 ½ cups button mushrooms
- 100 g / 3 ½ oz / 1 ½ cups sugar snap peas
- 50 ml / 1 ¾ fl. oz / ¼ cup vegetable stock
- salt and freshly ground black pepper

Method

1. Brush the turkey with half the oil, then sprinkle with thyme and season with salt and pepper.

2. Heat the rest of the oil in a frying pan and fry the lardons and onions for 10 minutes or until golden brown.

3. Meanwhile, heat a griddle pan until smoking hot. Griddle the turkey for 4 minutes on each side or until cooked through and nicely marked. Keep warm while you finish the vegetables.

4. Add the mushrooms and sugar snap peas to the lardon pan and stir-fry for 2 minutes, then pour in the vegetable stock and cover with a lid.

5. Steam with the lid on for 5 minutes, then season with salt and pepper. Cut each escalope in half and serve with the vegetables.

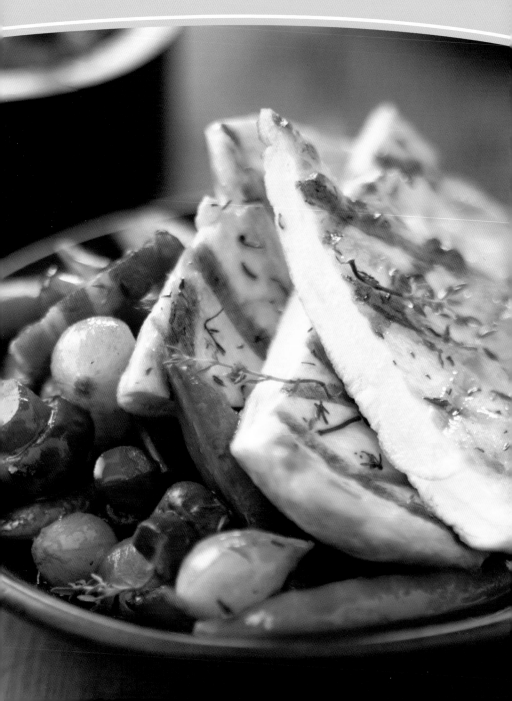

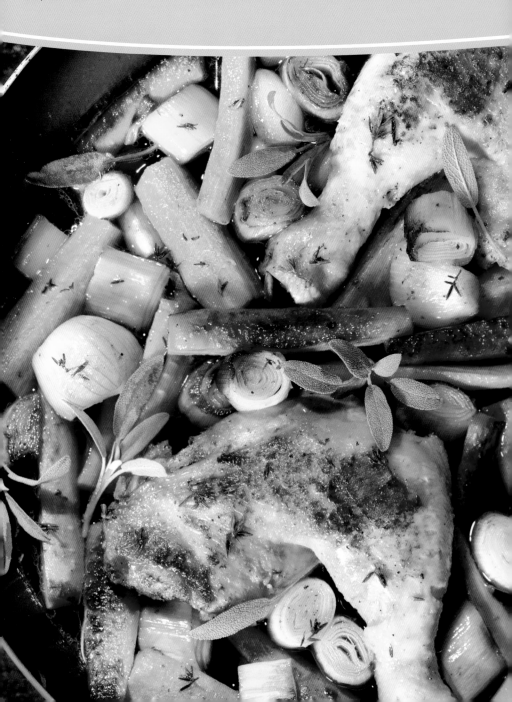

Sage and Honey Chicken

Serves: **4** | Preparation time: **5 minutes**
Cooking time: **50 minutes** | Calories per portion: **350**

Ingredients

- 2 x 200 g / 7 oz chicken leg quarters, skin-on
- 300 g / 10 ½ oz / 1 cup carrots, peeled and cut into batons
- 2 leeks, sliced
- 2 tbsp olive oil
- 1 tbsp fresh thyme leaves
- a few sprigs of sage, plus extra for garnishing
- 1 tbsp runny honey
- 1 tbsp cider vinegar
- salt and freshly ground black pepper

Method

1. Preheat the oven to 200°C (180°C fan) / 400F / gas 6. Arrange the chicken, carrots and leeks in a roasting tin, then drizzle with olive oil and massage it in.

2. Season with salt and pepper and sprinkle with thyme and sage, then bake for 45 minutes, stirring the vegetables occasionally.

3. Stir the honey into the vinegar and pour it over the chicken and vegetables, then return the tin to the oven for 5 minutes or until the honey starts to caramelise and the chicken is cooked through.

4. Divide each chicken quarter into a thigh and a leg and serve one piece of chicken per person with a quarter of the vegetables. Garnish with extra sage.

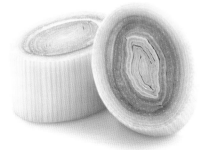

Steak Skewers

Serves: **4** | Preparation time: **2 hours**
Cooking time: **8 minutes** | Calories per portion: **211**

Ingredients

- 450 g / 1 lb sirloin steak, trimmed of fat
- ¼ yellow pepper
- ¼ red pepper
- ½ small courgette (zucchini)
- 4 salad onions, peeled
- a few sprigs of rosemary
- 2 tbsp olive oil
- 1 tbsp cider vinegar
- salt and freshly ground black pepper

Method

1. Cut the steak, peppers and courgette into large chunks and season with salt and pepper.

2. Tip them into a large sandwich bag with the salad onions and rosemary, then drizzle in the oil and vinegar. Seal the bag and leave to marinate for 2 hours.

3. Preheat the grill to its highest setting. Thread the meat and vegetables onto four metal skewers.

4. Cook the skewers under the grill for 8 minutes, turning occasionally, or until the vegetables are tender and the steak is nicely browned.

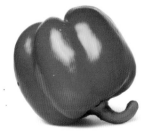
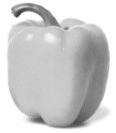

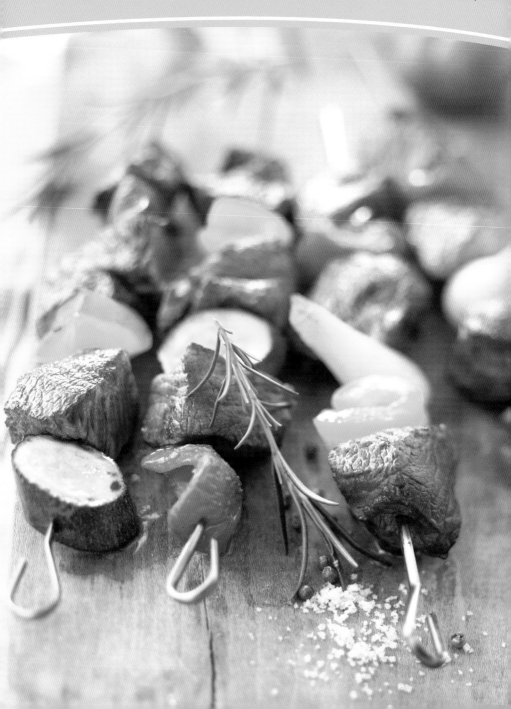

Chicken Satay Noodles

Serves: **4** | Preparation time: **5 minutes**
Cooking time: **30 minutes** | Calories per portion: **415**

Ingredients

- 200 g / 7 oz skinless chicken breast
- ½ aubergine (eggplant), cubed
- 1 courgette (zucchini), cut into chunks
- 1 medium carrot, cut into batons
- 8 asparagus spears, cut into short lengths
- 8 spring onions (scallions), cut into short lengths
- 8 baby corn cobs
- 1 tbsp sunflower oil
- 250 g / 9 oz / 1 ½ cups dried medium egg noodles
- a few sprigs of coriander (cilantro) to garnish
- salt and freshly ground black pepper

For the satay sauce:

- 2 tsp runny honey
- 4 tbsp crunchy peanut butter
- 2 tbsp lime juice
- 2 tbsp light soy sauce

Method

1. Preheat the oven to 190°C (170°C fan) / 375F / gas 5. Cut the chicken into strips and arrange in a roasting tin with the vegetables.

2. Drizzle over the oil then season with salt and pepper. Bake for 25 minutes or until the chicken is cooked through and the vegetables are tender, stirring occasionally.

3. Meanwhile, make the sauce by stirring all the ingredients together.

4. Towards the end of the chicken cooking time, boil a saucepan of water, then submerge the noodles, turn off the heat and leave to soften for 5 minutes.

5. Drain the noodles and toss with the chicken and vegetables. Divide between 4 bowls, drizzle with the satay sauce and garnish with coriander.

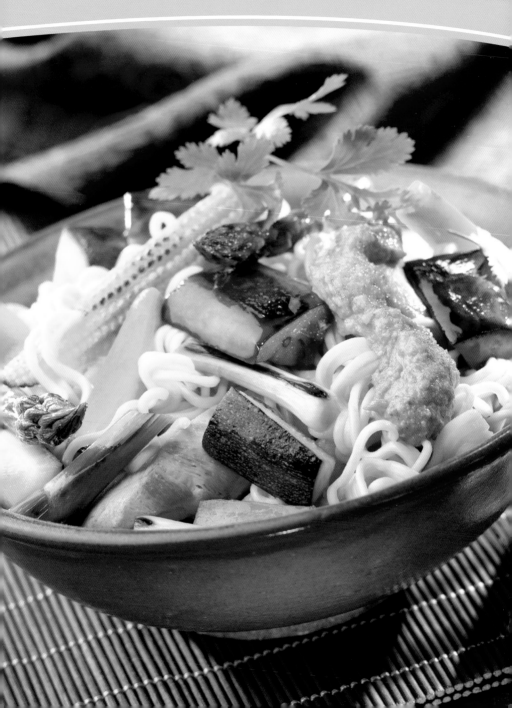

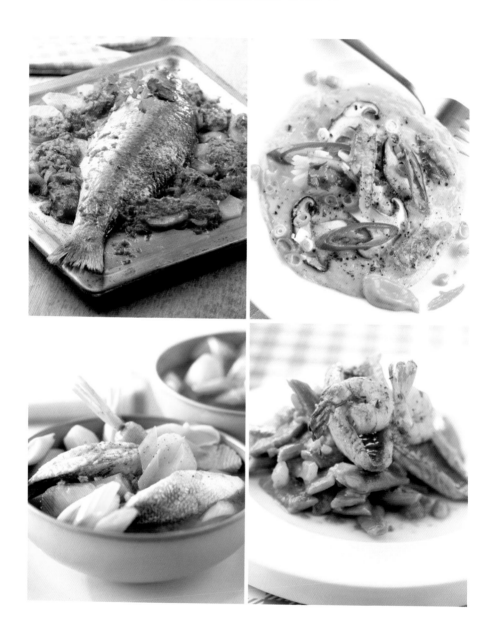

Fish

Including fish on your fast days is an excellent choice. Fish offers a high-protein addition to any meal and many types of fish are very low in calories. Always ensure that any fish you use is skinless. Some types of oily fish, such as salmon and tuna are also very high in essential oils.

Fish is a versatile ingredient that can be cooked in many ways – from steaming, baking and poaching to grilling. It's a handy part of the 5:2 diet as it's super-speedy to cook. That means even on a really busy day when you're pushed for time, you'll still be able to enjoy these recipes.

Mediterranean Sea Bass

Serves: **4** | Preparation time: **10 minutes**
Cooking time: **40 minutes** | Calories per portion: **419**

Ingredients

- 400 g / 14 oz / 2 cups potatoes, peeled and thickly sliced
- 900 g / 2 lb whole sea bass, gutted and scaled
- 1 onion, thinly sliced
- 190 g / 6 ½ oz / 1 cup red pepper pesto
- a few sprigs of flat leaf parsley to garnish

Method

1. Preheat the oven to 220°C (200°C fan) / 425F / gas 7. Boil the potatoes in salted water for 10 minutes, then drain well.
2. Spread out the potatoes on a baking tray and lay the sea bass on top.
3. Mix the onion with the pesto and spoon it over the potatoes and fish.
4. Transfer the baking tray to the oven and roast for 30 minutes or until the flesh of the bass comes away easily from the bone. If it starts to brown too quickly, cover the tray with foil.
5. Garnish with parsley and serve immediately.

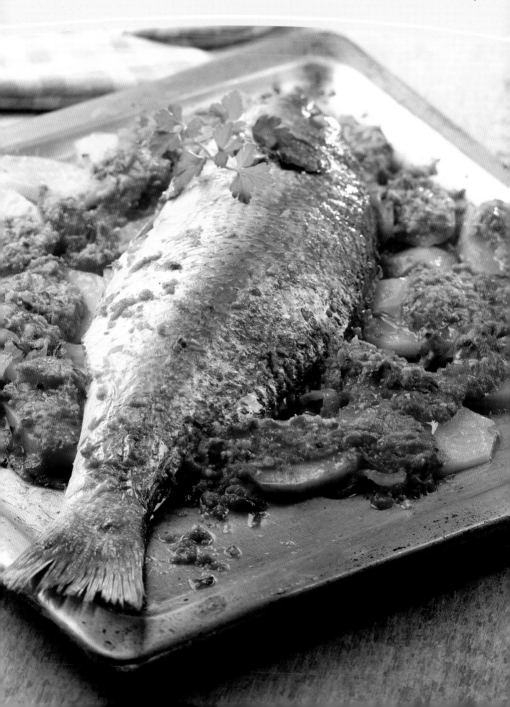

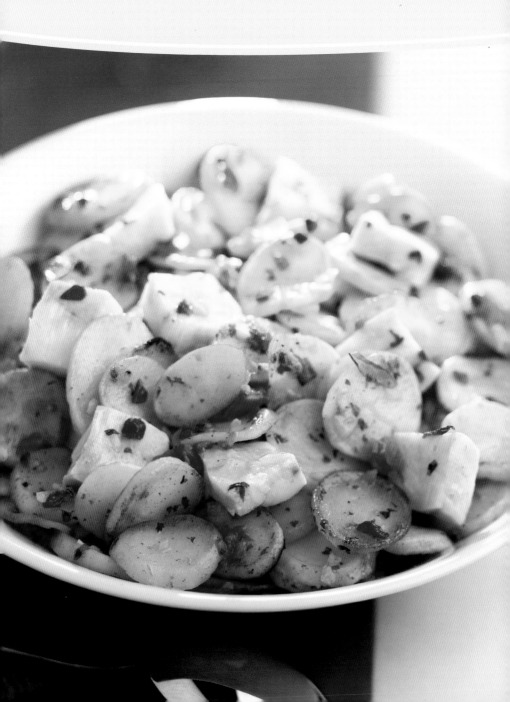

Spiced Cod and Potatoes

Serves: **2** | Preparation time: **10 minutes**
Cooking time: **45 minutes** | Calories per portion: **326**

Ingredients

- 300 g / 10 ½ oz / 2 cups new potatoes, sliced
- 1 shallot, chopped
- 2 cloves of garlic, chopped
- 2 long red chillies (chilies), deseeded and chopped
- 1 tbsp fresh oregano leaves
- 2 tbsp olive oil
- 150 g / 5 ½ oz piece of cod fillet
- salt and freshly ground black pepper

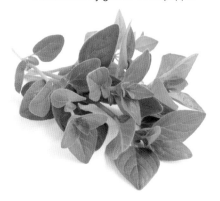

Method

1. Preheat the oven to 200°C (180° fan) / 400F / gas 6. Boil the potatoes in salted water for 10 minutes, then drain well.

2. While the potatoes are cooking, pound the shallot, garlic, chillies and oregano with a pestle and mortar. Stir in the oil to make a paste and season well with salt and pepper.

3. Spread out the potatoes in a roasting tin and massage in the spice paste.

4. Transfer the tin to the oven and roast for 20 minutes. Stir the potatoes, then position the cod on top and return to the oven for 15 minutes.

5. Flake the cod and stir it through the potatoes before serving.

Chilli Crab Omelette

Serves: **1** | Preparation time: **2 minutes**
Cooking time: **6 minutes** | Calories per portion: **224**

Ingredients

- 1 tsp olive oil
- 1 large egg, beaten
- 1 shitake mushroom, sliced
- 1 spring onion (scallion), sliced
- 50 g / 1 ¾ oz / ⅛ cup cooked white crab meat
- 1 tbsp sweet chilli (chili) sauce
- 1 long red chilli (chili), deseeded and sliced
- 1 tsp cooked brown crab meat
- 1 tsp light mayonnaise
- freshly ground black pepper

Method

1. Heat the oil in a small frying pan, then pour in the egg.

2. Arrange the mushroom, spring onion and white crab meat on top. Spoon over the chilli sauce and scatter over the chilli, then season well with black pepper.

3. When the egg has just set on top, slide the omelette onto a plate.

4. Stir the brown crab meat into the mayonnaise to make a smooth sauce and spoon onto the side of the plate.

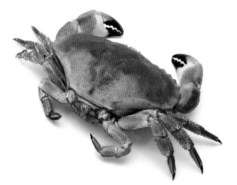

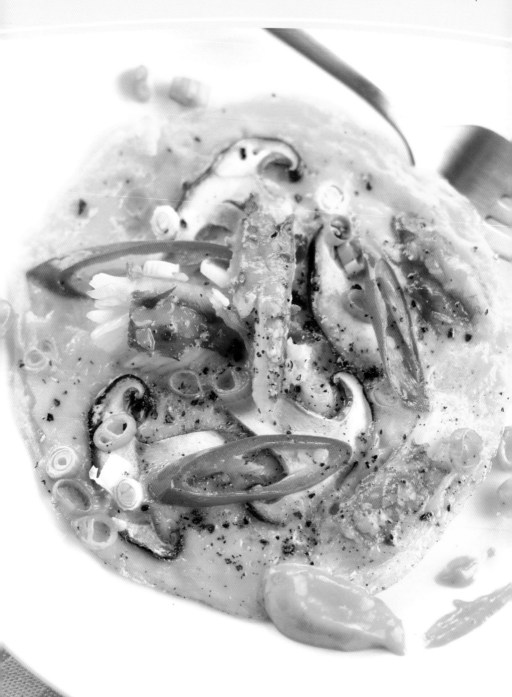

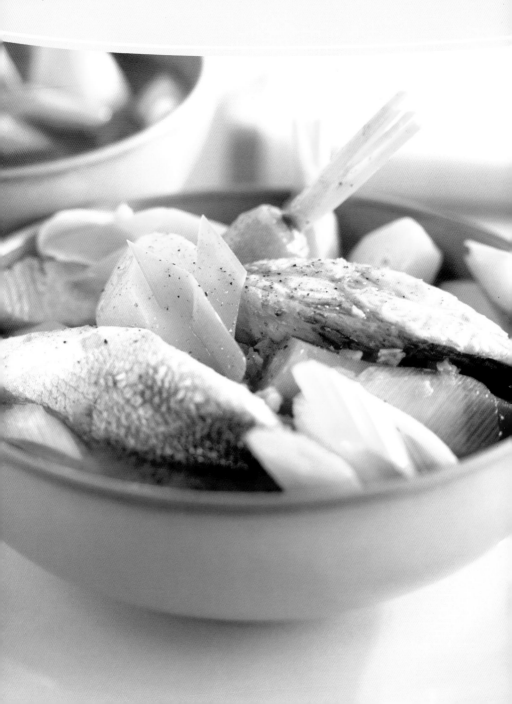

Light Fish Stew

Serves: **2** | Preparation time: **35 minutes**
Cooking time: **15 minutes** | Calories per portion: **313**

Ingredients

- 100 g / 3 ½ oz salmon fillet, skinned
- 250 g / 9 oz sea bass, gutted and scaled
- 1 clove of garlic, crushed
- 2 tbsp lemon juice
- 1 l / 1 pt 14 fl. oz / 4 cups vegetable or fish stock
- 100 g / 3 ½ oz / ⅔ cup new potatoes, peeled
- 100 g / 3 ½ oz / ¾ cup small carrots, peeled
- 1 leek, sliced
- salt and freshly ground black pepper

Method

1. Cut the salmon fillet into two equal pieces and cut the bass across into four steaks. Mix the garlic with the lemon juice and a pinch of salt and pepper, then pour it over the fish and leave to marinate for 30 minutes.

2. Pour the stock into a saucepan and set it over a high heat. When it starts to boil, add the potatoes, carrots and leeks and simmer for 10 minutes or until just tender.

3. Add the fish to the pan and poach gently for 4 minutes or until the flesh turns opaque.

4. Ladle into two warm bowls and serve immediately.

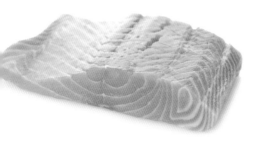

Provençal Mullet

Serves: **2** | Preparation time: **5 minutes**

Cooking time: **25 minutes** | Calories per portion: **400**

Ingredients

- 4 red mullet fillets
- 4 raw king prawns, peeled with tails left intact
- 2 tbsp olive oil
- ½ tsp smoked paprika
- 300 g / 10 ½ oz / 3 cups runner beans, cut into short lengths
- 1 onion, chopped
- 3 cloves of garlic, crushed
- 50 ml / 1 ¾ fl. oz / ¼ cup white wine
- 200 g / 7 oz / ¾ cup tomatoes, chopped
- 2 tsp flat leaf parsley, finely chopped
- salt

Method

1. Rub the mullet and prawns with half the oil and sprinkle with the paprika and salt.
2. Boil the beans for 4 minutes, then drain well and refresh in cold water.
3. Heat the rest of the oil in a saucepan and fry the onion and garlic over a low heat for 5 minutes. Increase the heat and pour in the wine, then reduce until almost evaporated.
4. Stir in the tomatoes and simmer for 5 minutes, then add the bean mixture and cook for a further 3 minutes.
5. Meanwhile, cook the mullet and prawns under a hot grill for 2 minutes on each side.
6. Divide the beans between two warm plates and top with the mullet, prawns and a sprinkle of parsley.

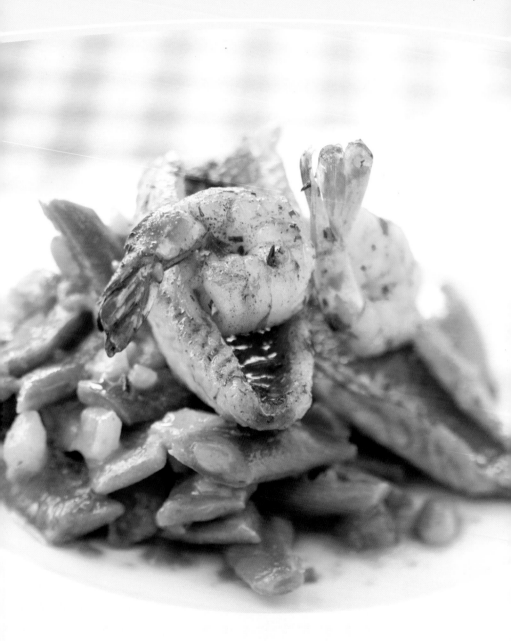

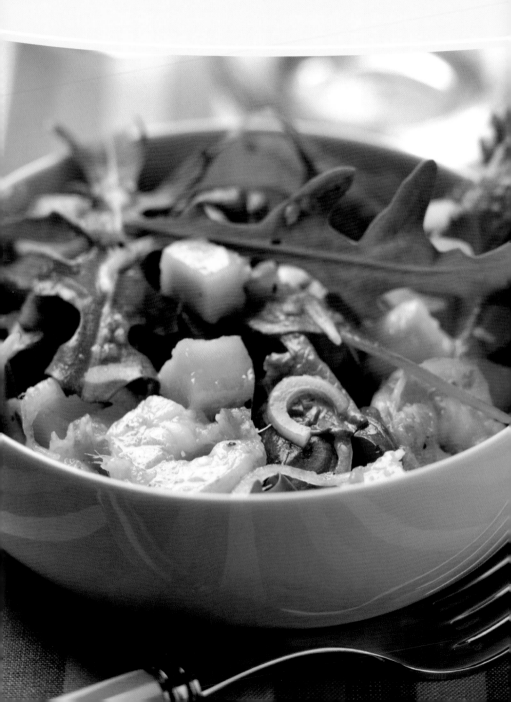

Prawn and Mango Salad

Serves: **1** | Preparation time: **15 minutes**
Calories per portion: **167**

Ingredients

- 1 tbsp caster (superfine) sugar
- 2 tbsp lime juice
- 1 tbsp fish sauce
- 1 tsp root ginger, finely grated
- 1 clove of garlic, crushed
- 1 shallot, sliced
- ½ medium mango, peeled and stoned
- 100 g / 3 ½ oz / ½ cup cooked king prawns, peeled
- 50 g / 1 ¾ oz / 2 cups rocket (arugula) leaves

Method

1. First make the dressing. Stir the sugar into the lime juice until it dissolves, then stir in the fish sauce, ginger, garlic and shallot. Leave to macerate for 10 minutes.

2. Cut the mango into small chunks, then toss with the prawns and rocket.

3. Drizzle over the dressing and serve immediately.

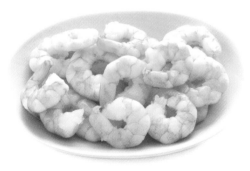

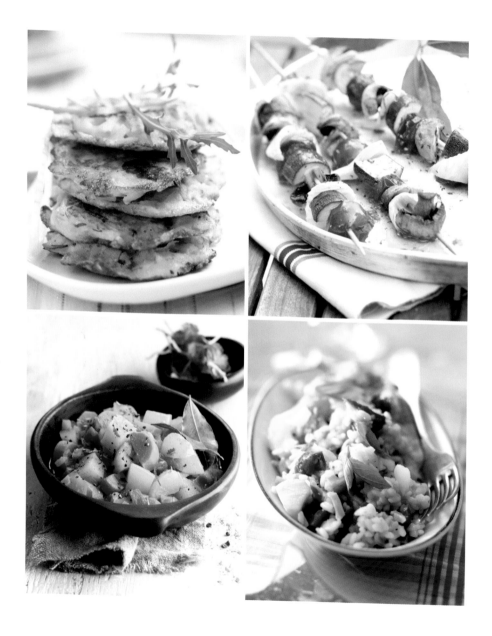

Vegetables

Like salads, vegetables can be a fast day's best buddy. High fibre, packed with vitamins and minerals and really filling, a good dollop of veg can go a long way to helping you feel full on 500-calorie days.

We've included a whole rainbow of veggie options in the next few pages, from good old vegetable stews to stir-fries and grilled options. The 5:2 diet is a great time to experiment with vegetables you've never tried before. Wander around the produce section of your supermarket and see what you can find!

Szechuan Stir-fry

Serves: **4** | Preparation time: **5 minutes**
Cooking time: **8 minutes** | Calories per portion: **119**

Ingredients

- 2 tbsp sunflower oil
- ½ tsp dried chilli (chili) flakes
- 1 tsp Szechuan peppercorns
- 100 g / 3 ½ oz / 1 ½ cups broccoli florets
- 8 asparagus spears, cut into short lengths
- 12 baby corn cobs
- 1 courgette (zucchini), cut into batons
- 8 spring onions (scallions), cut into short lengths
- 1 yellow and 1 red pepper, deseeded and sliced
- 2 tbsp light soy sauce

Method

1. Heat the oil in a large wok, then add the chilli and Szechuan peppercorns and stir-fry for 30 seconds.

2. Add the broccoli, asparagus and baby corn and stir-fry for 3 minutes.

3. Add the courgette, spring onions and peppers and stir-fry for a further 3 minutes.

4. Pour in the soy sauce and stir once, then put on the lid and steam for 1 minute.

5. Divide between four warm bowls and serve immediately.

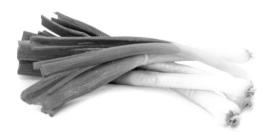

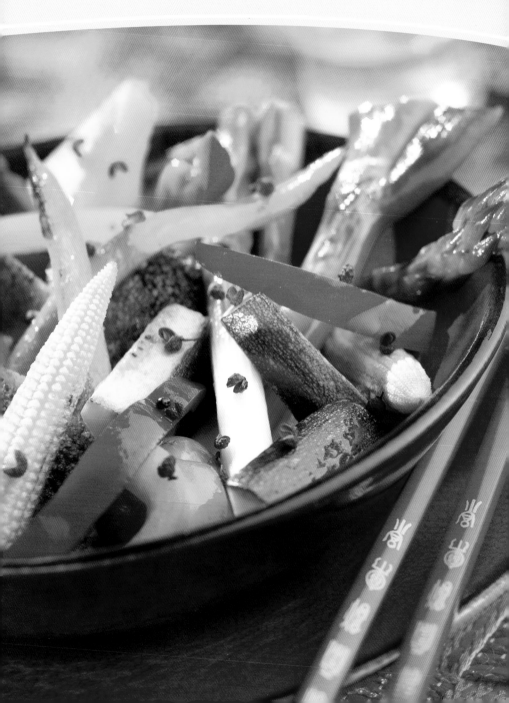

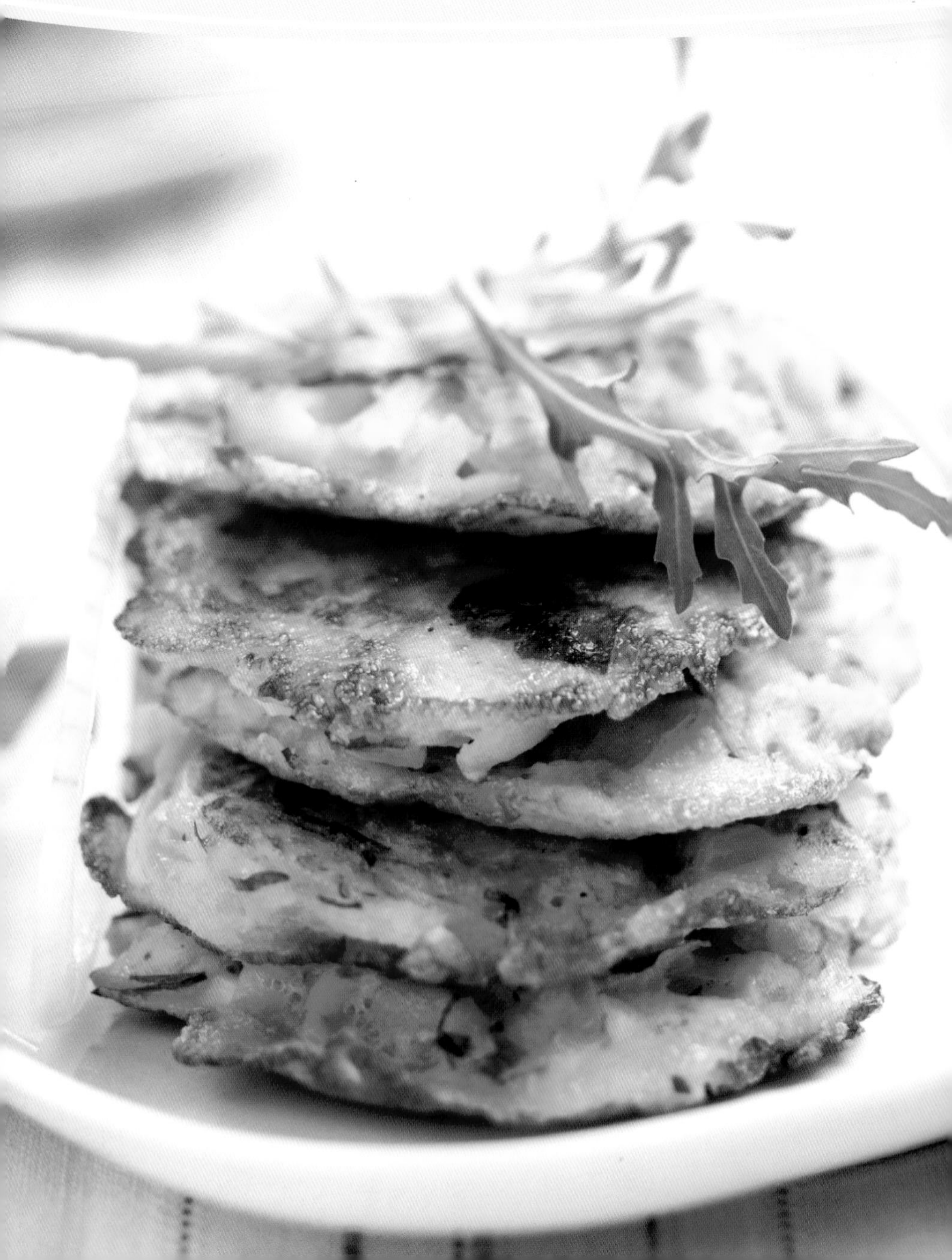

Healthy Potato Rosti

Serves: **2** | Preparation time: **1 hour 30 minutes**

Cooking time: **45 minutes** | Calories per portion: **149**

Ingredients

- 400 g / 14 oz / 2 ½ cups waxy potatoes
- 1 shallot, thinly sliced
- 1 tbsp French tarragon, roughly chopped
- 1 tsp Dijon mustard
- 1 large egg white
- 24 sprays of 1-cal olive oil spray
- salt and freshly ground black pepper

Method

1. Cook the unpeeled potatoes in boiling water for 18 minutes or until a skewer slides in easily. Drain well, then leave to cool completely before peeling.

2. Coarsely grate the potatoes and mix with the shallot and tarragon.

3. Whisk the mustard into the egg white and season with salt and pepper, then stir it into the potatoes. Shape the mixture into 6 flat patties then chill for 30 minutes.

4. Preheat the oven to 200°C (180°C fan) / 400F / gas 6. Line a baking tray with a non-stick baking mat. Carefully transfer the rostis to the tray and spray the top of each one with 4 sprays of oil.

5. Bake the rostis for 25 minutes or until golden brown.

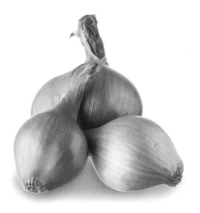

Vegetable Skewers

Serves: **4** | Preparation time: **1 hour**
Cooking time: **8 minutes** | Calories per portion: **95**

Ingredients

- 2 tbsp olive oil
- 1 tbsp cider vinegar
- 1 tsp dried herbs de Provence
- 1 courgette (zucchini), cut into chunks
- 18 cherry tomatoes, halved
- 12 button mushrooms, halved
- ½ fennel bulb, cut into chunks
- salt and freshly ground black pepper

Method

1. Mix the oil with the vinegar, herbs and a pinch of salt and pepper. Pour the mixture over the vegetables and leave to marinate for 1 hour.

2. Meanwhile, soak 12 wooden skewers in a bowl of cold water.

3. Preheat the grill to its highest setting. Thread the vegetables onto the skewers.

4. Cook the kebabs under the grill for 8 minutes, turning occasionally, or until the vegetables are tender and lightly toasted round the edges.

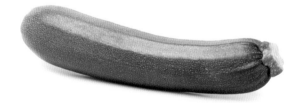

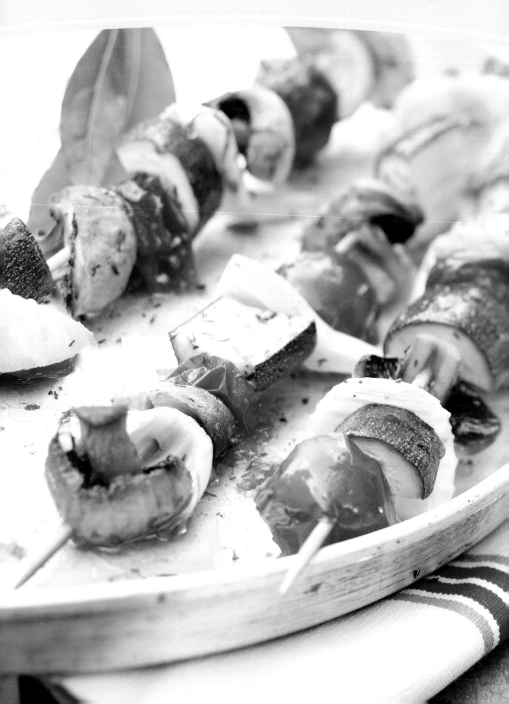

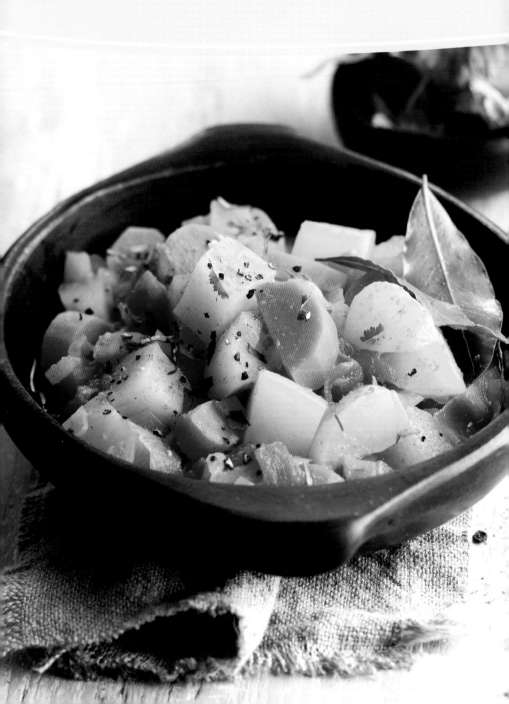

Spiced Vegetable Stew

Serves: **2** | Preparation time: **5 minutes**
Cooking time: **40 minutes** | Calories per portion: **225**

Ingredients

- 1 tbsp olive oil
- 1 onion, chopped
- 1 clove of garlic, crushed
- 2 bay leaves
- ½ tsp each ground coriander (cilantro) and turmeric
- 200 g / 7 oz / 1 ½ cups carrots, peeled and cut into chunks
- 200 g / 7 / 1 ⅓ cups potatoes, peeled and cut into chunks
- 400 g / 14 oz / 1 ⅔ cups canned tomatoes, chopped
- 250 ml / 9 fl. oz / 1 cup vegetable stock
- 1 tbsp coriander (cilantro) leaves, chopped
- salt and freshly ground black pepper

Method

1. Heat the oil in a saucepan and fry the onion and garlic for 5 minutes to soften.

2. Add the bay leaves, coriander and turmeric and stir well, then stir in the carrots and potatoes.

3. Pour in the chopped tomatoes and stock and simmer for 30 minutes or until the sauce has reduced and the vegetables are tender.

4. Season to taste with salt and freshly ground black pepper, then serve sprinkled with the coriander.

Artichoke Risotto

Serves: **2** | Preparation time: **5 minutes**
Cooking time: **35 minutes** | Calories per portion: **465**

Ingredients

- 500 ml / 17 ½ fl. oz / 2 cups vegetable stock
- 250 ml / 9 fl. oz / 1 cup skimmed milk
- 1 onion, finely chopped
- 3 cloves of garlic, crushed
- 1 tbsp olive oil
- 150 g / 5 ½ oz / 1 cup risotto rice
- 250 g / 5 ½ oz / 1 ½ cups canned artichoke hearts, drained and cubed
- 6 sun-dried tomatoes in oil, drained and chopped
- basil leaves to garnish
- salt and freshly ground black pepper

Method

1. Put the stock and milk in a saucepan and heat while you make the risotto base.

2. Fry the onion and garlic gently in the oil for 6 minutes without browning. Add the risotto rice and stir well to coat in the juices.

3. Add two ladles of the milky stock and let it bubble, stirring occasionally, until a trench drawn with the spoon doesn't immediately fill up with liquid.

4. Repeat with the rest of the stock, adding two ladles at a time, until the rice is just tender. Season with salt and pepper.

5. Stir in the artichokes and tomatoes, then cover the pan, turn off the heat and leave to stand for 5 minutes. Serve garnished with the basil.

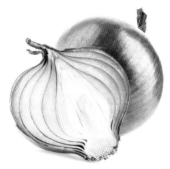

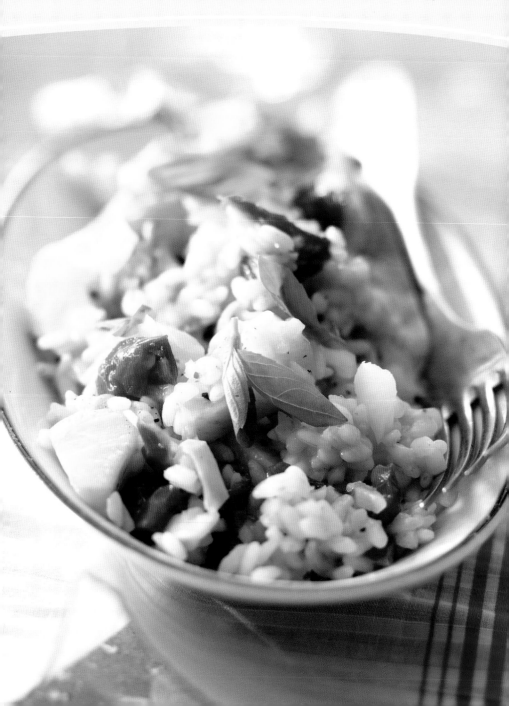

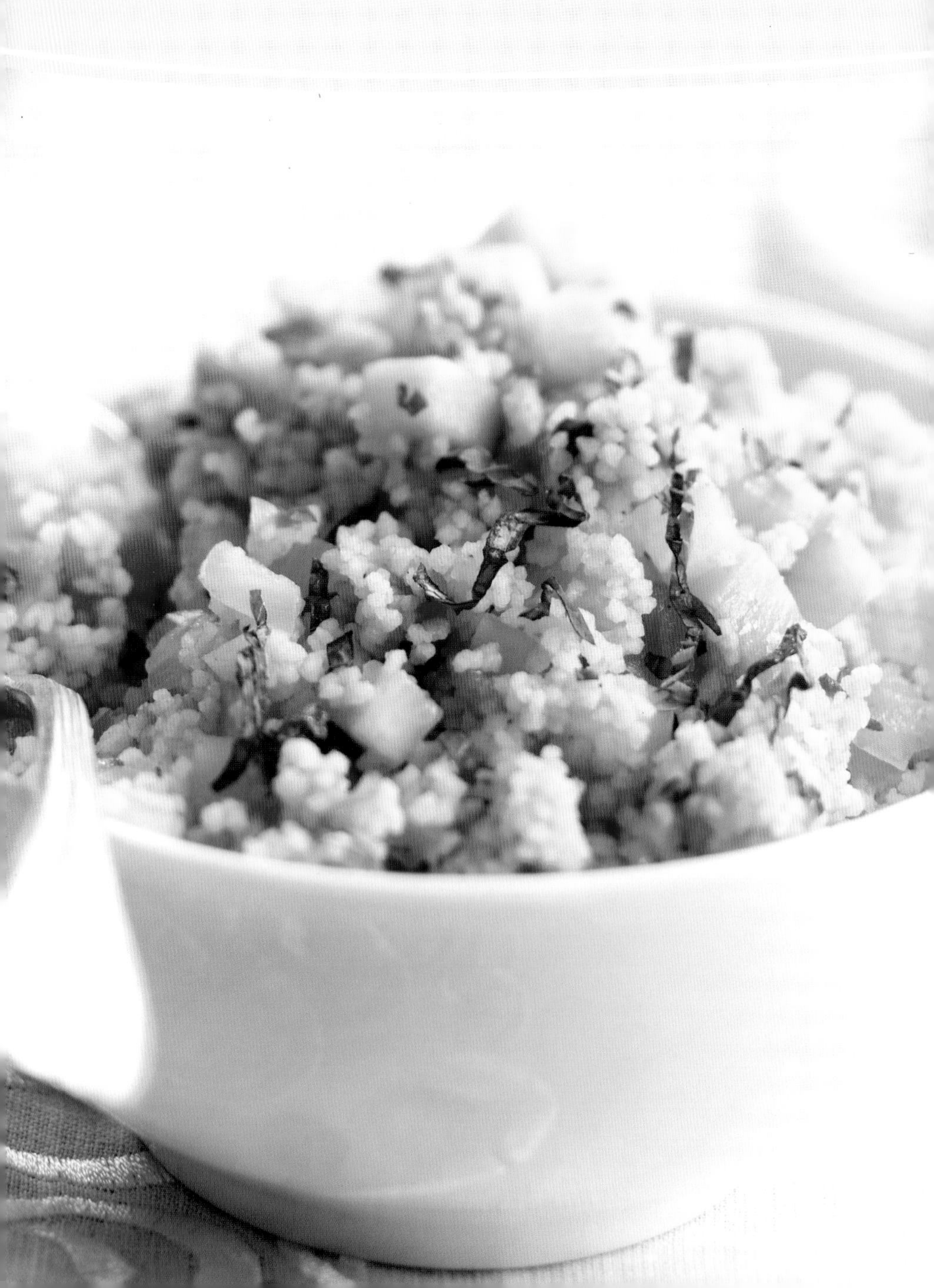

Couscous Salad

Serves: **4** | Preparation time: **2 minutes**
Cooking time: **5 minutes** | Calories per portion: **186**

Ingredients

- 180 g / 6 oz / 1 cup couscous
- ½ medium cucumber, diced
- 2 tomatoes, finely chopped
- ½ onion, finely chopped
- 1 tbsp mint leaves, shredded
- 1 tbsp basil leaves, shredded
- 2 tbsp lemon juice
- salt

Method

1. Put the couscous in a bowl with a big pinch of salt and pour over 290 ml of boiling water. Cover the bowl tightly with cling film and leave to stand for 5 minutes.

2. When the time is up, fluff up the grains with a fork and stir through the vegetables, herbs and lemon juice.

3. Serve warm straight away or chill in the fridge and serve cold.

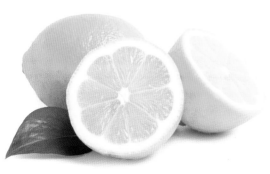

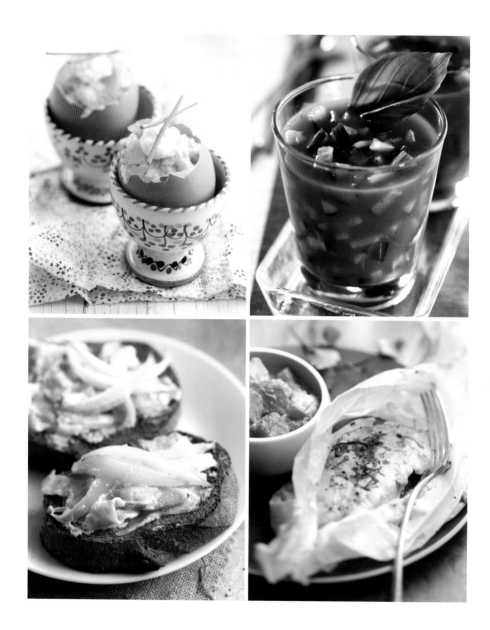

Supper

If you're the sort of person to save up most of your calories for the evening, then supper will be right up your street. This early evening meal can feel like a reward for sticking to your calorie limit so carefully throughout the day.

Our supper recipes have something for everyone, from good old favourites and fresh seasonal meals to winter warming recipes. Don't forget to pep up your plate with additional low calorie vegetables (such as cabbage and broccoli) or add a salad plate of fresh leaves with herbs.

Smoked Salmon Scramble

Serves: **1** | Preparation time: **5 minutes**
Cooking time: **4 minutes** | Calories per portion: **191**

Ingredients

- 2 large eggs
- 25 g / 1 oz / ⅛ cup smoked salmon, chopped
- 1 tsp 0% fat Greek yoghurt
- 1 chive, cut into short lengths
- salt

Method

1. Break the eggs into a small saucepan, retaining the bigger half of the shells. Carefully rinse and dry the egg shells, then sit them inside 2 egg cups.

2. Gently beat the eggs in the saucepan with a pinch of salt.

3. Turn on the heat under the pan and stir the eggs until they scramble, then spoon them back into their shells.

4. Top each egg with smoked salmon and yoghurt, then garnish with chives before serving.

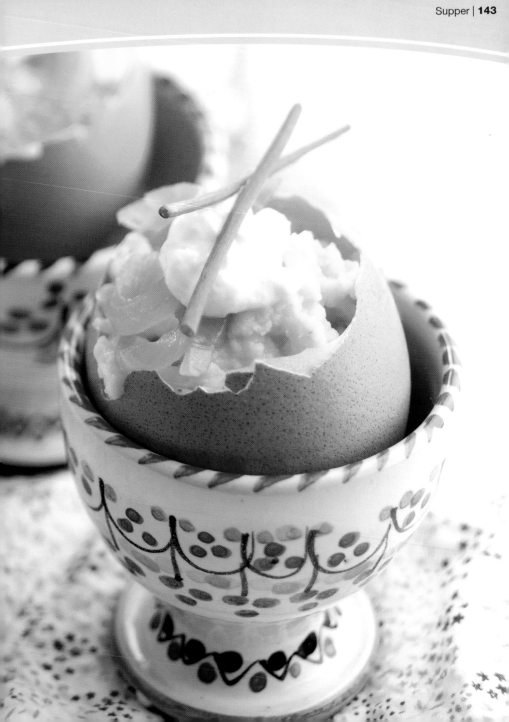

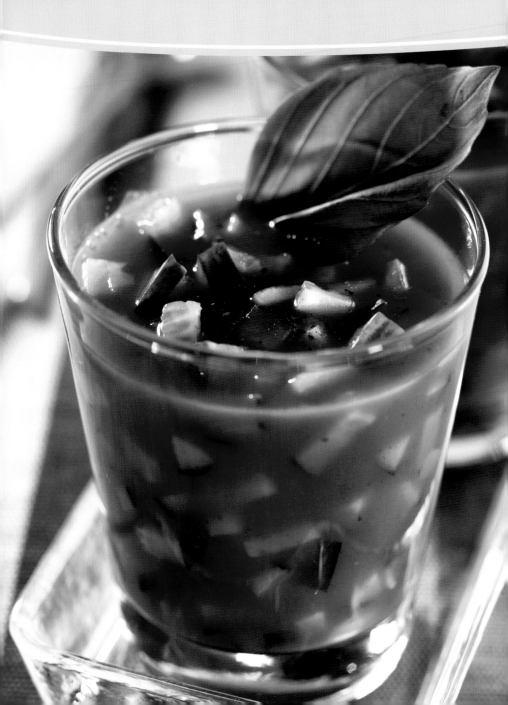

Gazpacho Soup

Serves: **4** | Preparation time: **5 minutes**
Calories per portion: **34**

Ingredients

- 1 medium cucumber, diced
- 2 spring onions (scallions), finely chopped
- 250 g / 9 oz / 1 cup ripe tomatoes, cubed
- 1 red pepper, diced
- 2 tbsp sherry vinegar
- 1 tbsp basil leaves, chopped, plus extra to garnish
- salt and freshly ground black pepper

Method

1. Put half of the cucumber in a liquidiser with the rest of the ingredients and blend until smooth.

2. Pass the mixture through a sieve then stir in the rest of the cucumber and season to taste with salt and pepper.

3. Serve garnished with the basil.

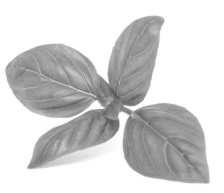

Alsace Toasts

Serves: **2** | Preparation time: **2 minutes**
Cooking time: **5 minutes** | Calories per portion: **143**

Ingredients

- 2 slices of baguette
- 1 tbsp low-fat soft cheese
- 2 rashers unsmoked back bacon, sliced
- ½ onion, sliced

Method

1. Toast the bread on one side under a hot grill.
2. Turn it over and spread the untoasted side with the cheese, then arrange the bacon and onion on top.
3. Put the bread back under the grill and cook until the bacon has turned opaque and the onions have softened.

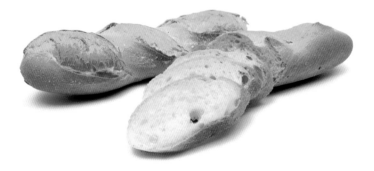

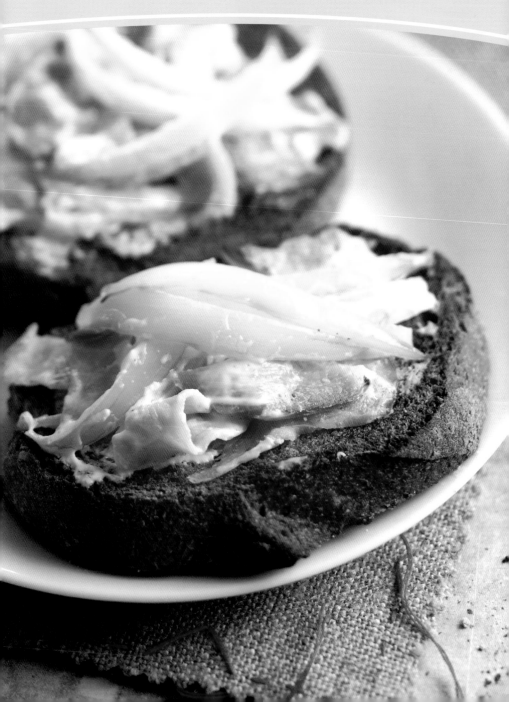

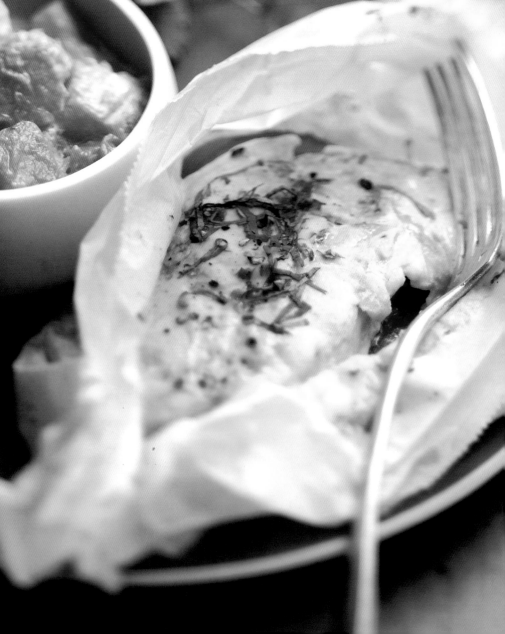

Sole en Papillote

Serves: **2** | Preparation time: **5 minutes**
Cooking time: **15 minutes** | Calories per portion: **250**

Ingredients

- 2 tomatoes, sliced
- 2 x 200 g fillets of sole, skinned
- 2 tsp Dijon mustard
- 1 tbsp basil leaves, shredded

For the sweet potatoes:

- 1 medium sweet potato, peeled and cubed
- 500 ml / 17 ½ fl. oz / 2 cups skimmed milk (calories not counted as discarded after use)
- salt and freshly ground black pepper

Method

1. Preheat the oven to 200°C (180°C fan) / 400F / gas 6.

2. Divide the tomatoes between 2 large sheets of baking parchment. Position the sole on top and spread with the mustard, then sprinkle with the basil and season with salt and pepper.

3. Fold over the parchment and twist the ends to seal, then transfer the parcels to a baking sheet. Bake in the oven for 15 minutes.

4. To prepare the sweet potatoes, put them in a deep saucepan with the milk and enough water to cover. Add 1 tsp of salt then boil for 15 minutes or until tender. Drain and discard the milk before serving with the sole.

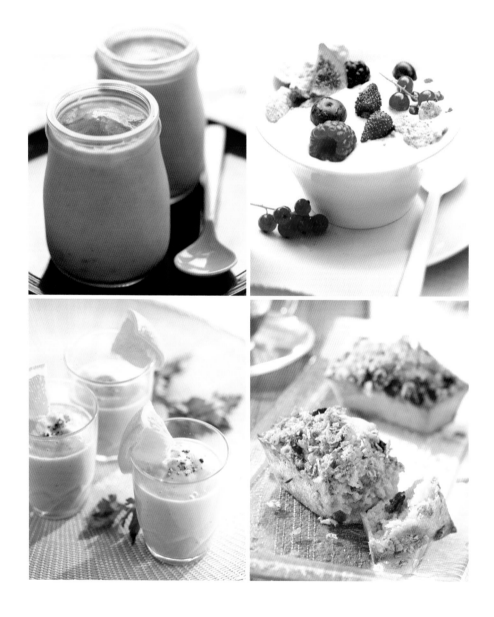

Snacks and Treats

The idea of having any snacks or treats at all on a fast day might seem no-go to you. But when you are severely restricting your calorie intake, the odd low-calorie snack can be all you need to keep you on the straight and narrow before you return to normal eating tomorrow.

We've included something for everyone here, from tempting treats for the sweet-toothed, to mouthwatering snacks for when you feel like something to munch. Many of them can be prepared in an instant – a quick way to stave off those cravings!

Blueberry Yoghurt

Serves: **2** | Preparation time: **2 minutes**
Calories per portion: **91**

Ingredients

- 150 g / 5 ½ oz / ¾ cup 0% fat Greek yoghurt
- 50 g / 1 ¾ oz / ⅓ cup blueberries
- 1 tbsp runny honey

Method

1. Put the yoghurt, berries and honey in a food processor and blend until smooth.
2. Spoon into two glass yoghurt pots and serve.

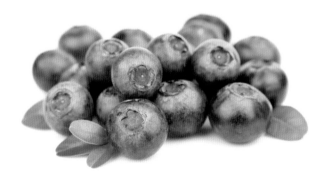

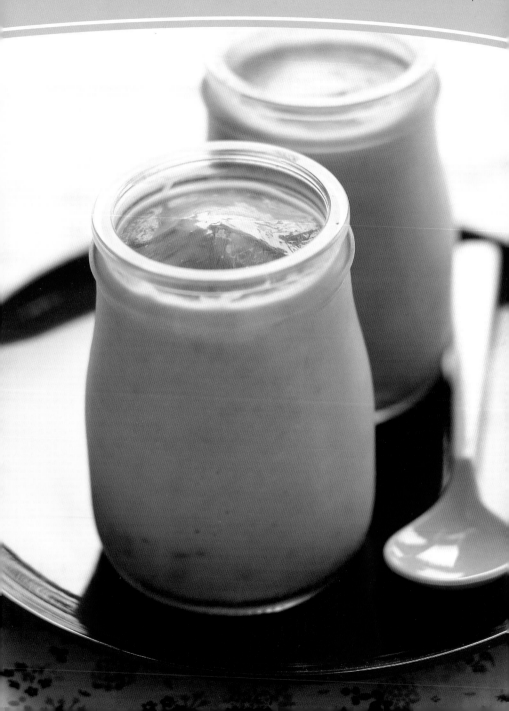

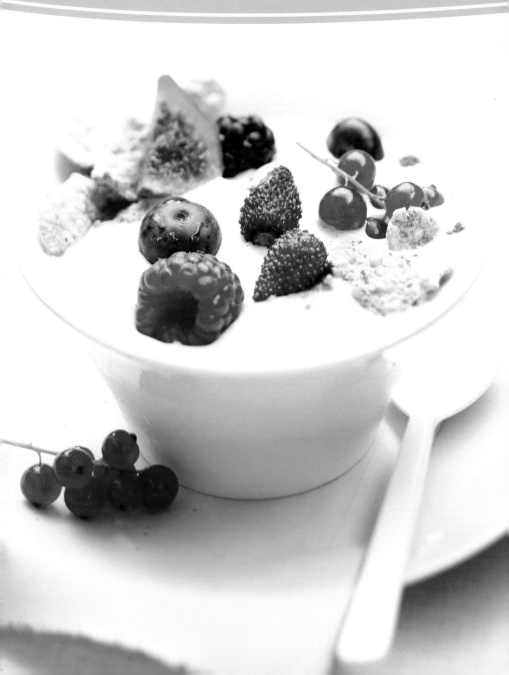

Fruity Fromage Frais

Serves: **2** | Preparation time: **2 minutes**
Calories per portion: **142**

Ingredients

- 1 tbsp runny honey
- 200 g / 7 oz / 1 cup 3.4% fat fromage frais
- 50 g / 1 ½ oz / ⅓ cup mixed summer fruit
- 2 tbsp wholegrain cereal flakes

Method

1. Stir the honey into the fromage frais and divide between two bowls.

2. Sprinkle over the fruit and cereal flakes, then serve straight away.

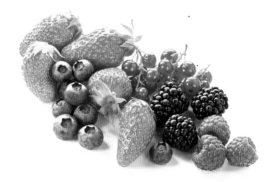

Avocado Smoothie

Serves: **4** | Preparation time: **5 minutes**
Calories per portion: **163**

Ingredients

- 1 ripe avocado, skinned, stoned and chopped
- 100 g / 3 ½ oz / ½ cup 0% fat Greek yoghurt
- 1 medium banana, sliced
- 2 navel oranges, juiced, plus extra wedges to decorate
- 1 tbsp runny honey

Method

1. Put all of the ingredients in a liquidiser and blend until smooth.

2. Pour into 4 glasses and serve garnished with orange wedges.

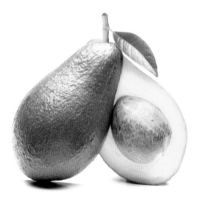

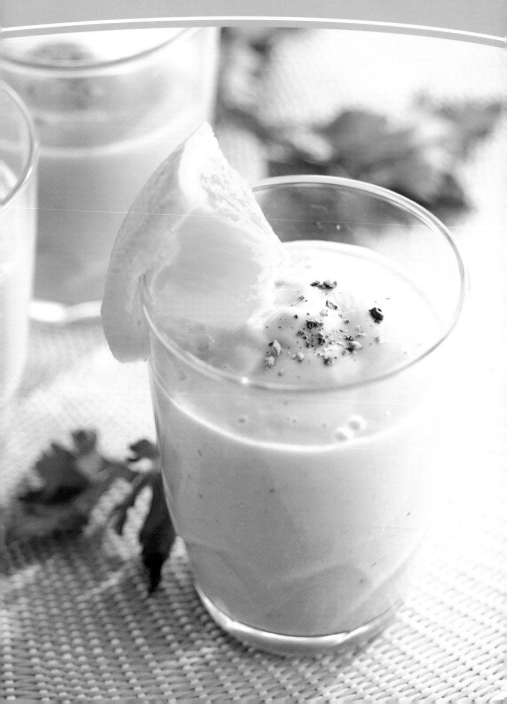

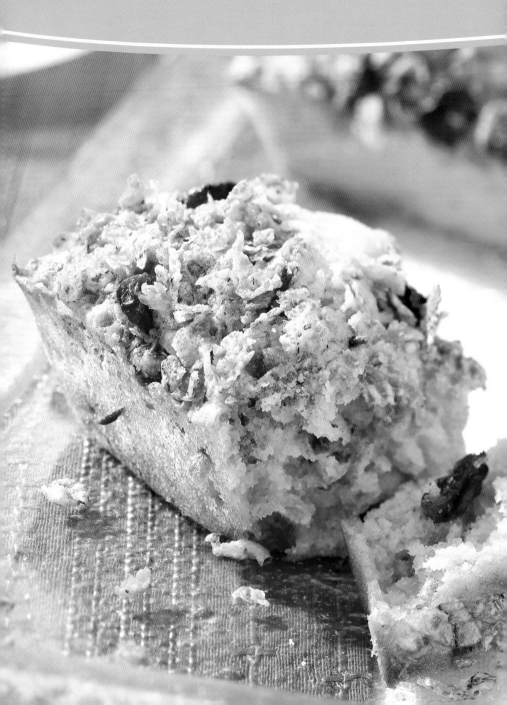

Muesli Cake Bars

Makes: **12** | Preparation time: **15 minutes**
Cooking time: **10–15 minutes** | Calories per portion: **123**

Ingredients

- 4 large eggs, separated
- 175 g / 6 oz / ¾ cup caster (superfine) sugar
- 50 g / 1 ¾ oz / ½ cup unsweetened muesli
- 100 g / 3 ½ oz / ⅔ cup self-raising flour

Method

1. Preheat the oven to 180°C (160°C fan) / 350F / gas 4 and oil a 12-hole silicone mini loaf cake mould.

2. Whisk the egg yolks and sugar together for 4 minutes or until pale and thick, then fold in the flour and half the muesli.

3. Whip the egg white to stiff peaks in a clean bowl, then fold it into the cake mixture in two stages.

4. Spoon the mixture into the mould and sprinkle with the rest of the muesli.

5. Bake for 10–15 minutes or until a skewer inserted comes out clean. Leave to cool in the mould for 10 minutes before transferring to a wire rack to cool completely.

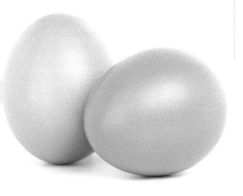

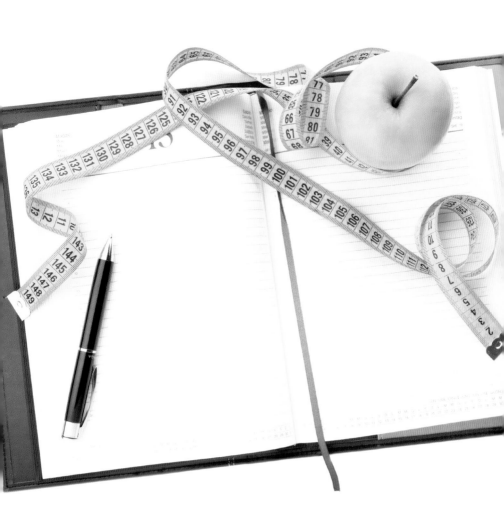

Dear Diary...

It's easy to lose track of what we eat on a daily basis and while you're trying to lose weight it's a good idea to jot down what you've eaten and when.

This not only helps you to stick to your 500-calorie limit on fast days but it also means you can spot days and times when keeping to the guidelines may be a little harder.

If you write things down, you simply can't 'forget' about that biscuit or that extra slice of ham you wolfed down while waiting for lunch to cook. Keeping a diary is especially important for the 5:2 diet as you'll be able to assess which days work best for you, and which meals help you to get through the two fast days. Keep a note of any exercise (both formal and informal) that you do, too.

Week 1

	Fast Day 1	Fast Day 2
Breakfast		
Lunch		
Dinner		
Snacks		
Exercise		
Total Cals		

Today I weigh

Weight loss so far

Fast days

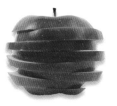

How I feel

Exercise log

top tip

Find a photograph of a celebrity whose figure you most admire and stick it on the inside of your kitchen cupboards for inspiration.

Week 2

	Fast Day 1	Fast Day 2
Breakfast		
Lunch		
Dinner		
Snacks		
Exercise		
Total Cals		

Today I weigh   *Fast days*

Weight loss so far

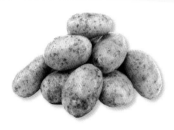

How I feel

Exercise log

Week 3

	Fast Day 1	Fast Day 2
Breakfast		
Lunch		
Dinner		
Snacks		
Exercise		
Total Cals		

Today I weigh

Fast days

Weight loss so far

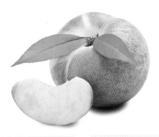

How I feel   Exercise log

Week 4

	Fast Day 1	Fast Day 2
Breakfast		
Lunch		
Dinner		
Snacks		
Exercise		
Total Cals		

Today I weigh   *Fast days*

Weight loss so far

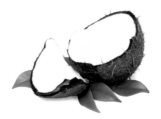

How I feel

Exercise log

top tip

Dig it! If you have a patch of land, give it the once over. Clearing a patch of soil can be quite a liberating experience. Even more exciting, you can think about what you're going to plant in the area. Flowers? Vegetables. This could be the start of grow-your-own!

Week 5

	Fast Day 1	Fast Day 2
Breakfast		
Lunch		
Dinner		
Snacks		
Exercise		
Total Cals		

Today I weigh

Fast days

Weight loss so far

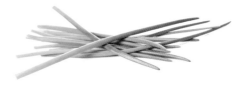

How I feel   Exercise log

top tip

**Find a weight-loss buddy
who's trying to shed a few
pounds too. That way you
can encourage each other
and swap recipes.**

Week 6

	Fast Day 1	Fast Day 2
Breakfast		
Lunch		
Dinner		
Snacks		
Exercise		
Total Cals		

Today I weigh

Weight loss so far

Fast days

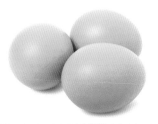

How I feel

Exercise log

top tip

Liven up your cold drinks by freezing low calorie squash and adding them to water. Mix and match. Imagine how tasty orange and blackcurrant ice cubes make that glass of water.

Week 7

	Fast Day 1	Fast Day 2
Breakfast		
Lunch		
Dinner		
Snacks		
Exercise		
Total Cals		

Today I weigh   *Fast days*

Weight loss so far

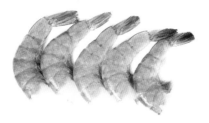

How I feel

Exercise log

top tip

Try a new exercise on top of all your daily activity. Look out for news of new classes on local notice boards. How about zumba or line dancing? Many of them are pay as you go so there's no need to sign up for a whole year.

Week 8

	Fast Day 1	Fast Day 2
Breakfast		
Lunch		
Dinner		
Snacks		
Exercise		
Total Cals		

Today I weigh

Fast days

Weight loss so far

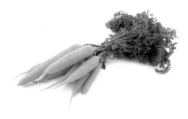

How I feel   Exercise log

top tip

Go to work on an egg. Incorporate an egg-based meal into one of your fast days this week. Eggs are wonderful little things – they're cheap, packed with protein and keep you feeling nice and full.

Week 9

	Fast Day 1	Fast Day 2
Breakfast		
Lunch		
Dinner		
Snacks		
Exercise		
Total Cals		

Today I weigh

Fast days

Weight loss so far

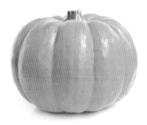

How I feel

Exercise log

top tip

Get merry with berries. Soft
fruits such as blackberries,
strawberries and raspberries
are all jam-packed with
vitamin C and fibre and
are very low in calories. If
you have a sweet craving,
pop open a box of frozen
raspberries and eat them
like sweets.

Week 10

	Fast Day 1	Fast Day 2
Breakfast		
Lunch		
Dinner		
Snacks		
Exercise		
Total Cals		

Today I weigh   *Fast days*

Weight loss so far

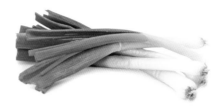

How I feel

Exercise log

top tip

**Get to the bottom of it.
Check out those feet. On a
fast day, to take your mind
off food, treat yourself to a
home pedicure. Exfoliate and
moisturise and then paint
those twinkling tootsies with
a dazzling nail polish. Ta-da!**

Week 11

	Fast Day 1	Fast Day 2
Breakfast		
Lunch		
Dinner		
Snacks		
Exercise		
Total Cals		

Today I weigh   *Fast days*

Weight loss so far

How I feel

Exercise log

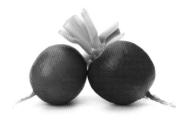

Week 12

	Fast Day 1	Fast Day 2
Breakfast		
Lunch		
Dinner		
Snacks		
Exercise		
Total Cals		

Today I weigh   *Fast days*

Weight loss so far

How I feel

Exercise log

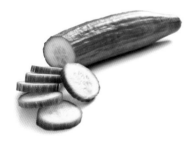

Staying Slim

Getting slim is one thing, now you want to be sure you can stay at your wonderful new weight. Many dieters gain the pounds back on because they revert to old eating habits and they start to get lazy about keeping active.

You don't want to undo all that hard work, do you? So here are a few tips to making sure that the new you becomes the always you.

• Rather than abandoning the whole 5:2 principle all together, why not go 6:1 and have six days of ordinary eating a week, allowing one day for a 500 calorie fast? Now that you're well used to fitting fasting days into your routine, you'll find this an easy way to maintain your new weight. Use your one fast day a week to revisit all the recipes that helped you through in the first place.

• Keep up the activity levels, rain or shine. No matter what the weather, keep up the brisk walks. They're great for toning, for boosting your mood and for putting a smile on your face.

• Remember!!! Yes, don't forget why you did the 5:2 diet in the first place. Keep an old picture of yourself next to one of your new slim self. You don't want to backtrack now, do you?

• If you've gone down a dress size – or two – then have a great big wardrobe clear out. Package up any clothes that are too large and either sell them at a car boot sale, on an auction site or – be generous and donate them to charity. Think how good that makes you feel!

• Incorporate some of the 5:2 recipes into everyday menus. They make a good balance on days when you've had a hefty lunch or are late getting up.

• Take the compliments. When people tell you how good you're looking, hold your head up and thank them. It's all too easy to dismiss it when someone says something nice to us. But go right ahead. Smile. You worked hard. You deserve the praise.

• Set an example. If you have children or young people in your life, let them see you enjoying fruits and vegetables, swooning over salads and crooning over cabbage. They'll soon see how happy and healthy eating a varied diet makes you feel.

• Keep track. Weigh yourself once a week and pat yourself on the back every time you maintain weight.

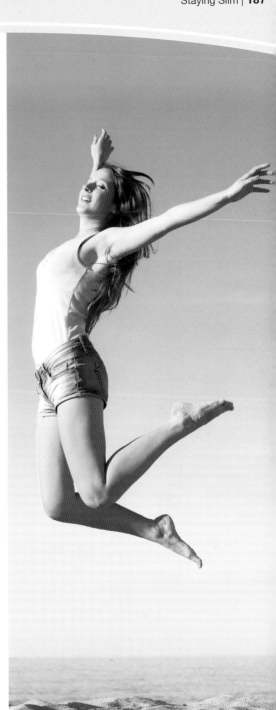

Notes

Notes

Notes

_____

_____

_____

_____

_____

_____

_____

_____

_____

_____

_____

_____

_____

_____

_____

_____

_____

_____

_____

_____

_____

_____

_____

Notes

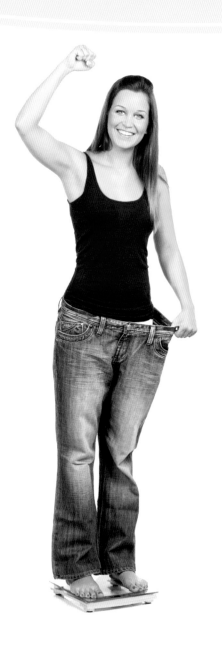

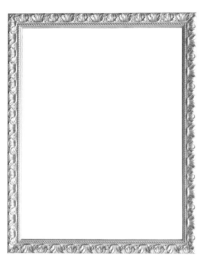

Before

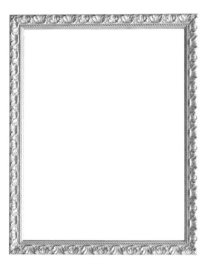

After